ARTHRITIS

Don't
Learn to Live
with It

BY

CARLTON
FREDERICKS,

Ph. D.

ARTHRITIS

Don't
Learn to Live
with It

BY

CARLTON
FREDERICKS,

Ph.D.

A Perigee Book

Perigee Books
are published by
The Putnam Publishing Group
200 Madison Avenue
New York, NY 10016

Library of Congress Cataloging in Publication Data

Fredericks, Carlton.
    Arthritis, don't learn to live with it.

    Reprint. Originally published: New York:
Grosset & Dunlap, c1981.
    Includes bibliographical references and index.
    1. Arthritis—Nutritional aspects.   2. Arthritis—
Diet therapy.   I. Title.
RC933.F718   1985   616.7'220654   84-18961
ISBN 0-399-51133-4

Printed in the United States of America

7   8   9   10

Contents

Aware that delay is the worst form of denial, and the deprivation most grievous for those with chronic disease, a small band of researchers braved the wrath of the establishment by investigating—and establishing—the value of nutrition in arthritis. I dedicate this book to them: Norman F. Childers, Ph.D., William Kaufman, M.D., John M. Ellis, M.D., Tom Spies, M.D., and the thousands of practitioners in holistic medicine who have applied their findings to help those who have been told that you take aspirin and learn to live with arthritis.

Carlton Fredericks, Ph.D, F.I.A.P.M.

An Author's Biography

Education: B.A., University of Alabama, 1931. M.A., 1949, and Ph. D., 1955, New York University, School of Education. Major: public health education. Dissertation: study of the responses of adults to nutrition education via a mass medium.

Teaching posts: Adult continuing education: City College of New York, Brooklyn College, Rockland Community College, New York Institute of Technology.

Faculty posts: New York University, School of Education, lecturer. Mercy College, professor. Fairleigh Dickinson, College of Education, professor (current position).

Subjects: nutrition for health supervisors, basic nutrition, nutrition for consultants, advanced (graduate) nutrition.

Visiting clinician: continuing education in nutrition for graduate dentists, University of California, Los Angeles, College of Dentistry. Honor panel, MidWinter Dental Clinic, Dallas Dental Society. Continuing nutrition education for physicians, International College of Applied Nutrition.

Societies: International Academy of Preventive Medicine, past president, honorary trustee, and fellow. American Academy of Medical Preventics, honorary president. International College of Applied Nutrition, founding fellow. International Academy Metabology, lifetime member. Academy of Orthomolecular Psychiatry, honorary fellow. American Institute of Stress, trustee. Price Pottenger Foun-

7

dation, fellow. International Foundation for BioSocial Development and Human Health, trustee. Society for the Protection of the Unborn Through Nutrition, member. Rio Hondo Area Drug Abuse Coalition, Advisory Board. *Honors:* Phi Beta Kappa. Mensa. Citations for services in nutrition education and research, from The Huxley Institute, the North Nassau Mental Health Center, the International Academy of Preventive Medicine, the Academy of Orthomolecular Psychiatry, the International Academy Metabology, and others. *Who's Who in the East*, 1979-80, and numerous other reference volumes.

An Introduction Which Is Required Reading

On occasion, detractors have pointed out that my ten books do not include a single text that is approved by the American Medical Association or the Harvard nutrition department. I have responded by suggesting that such approval would mean that I had failed in my responsibilities to the public, and would promptly rewrite any book that did obtain their endorsement. All this explains why I have preceded this Introduction with my complete educational and professional biography, for I am certain that the Arthritis Foundation will list this book, too, as "not recommended," although it is thoroughly documented from competent sources, and my training and experience in preventive and therapeutic nutrition have qualified me as an instructor for the professions. But history confirms that the Arthritis Foundation, which controls orthodox thinking in that field, has always approved a long list of toxic drugs for the treatment of the arthritic diseases, while flatly and totally rejecting poor nutrition as a cause of arthritis, and nutritional therapy as an effective treatment. So it is that nonhormonal anti-inflammation drugs are approved, though their dangers may and frequently do outweigh their benefits. Gold therapy draws no adverse comment, though it may depress the bone marrow or adversely affect eyesight. Aspirin is honored, despite its tendencies to cause gastric hemorrhaging and to interfere with the body's utilization of Vitamin C. Penicillamine treatment has official blessing, too, though in any group treated with it there is a large percentage for whom it does far more harm than good. Cortisone and other synthetic hormones are orthodox treatments, though the list of possible (and frequent) side reactions includes atrophy of the adrenal glands, retention of fluid, rises in blood pressure, decalcification of bones, gastric ulcer, and reduced resistance to infection. But any attempt to prevent or to treat arthritis with nutrition is considered quackery. The position of the orthodoxy is clear, which is more than can be said for its thinking: bad diet doesn't cause arthritis, and good nutrition doesn't help it. So it is that books on nutrition in arthritis will inevitably emerge on a black list.

As an arthritic who may have been told to take aspirin and learn to live with it, you may find it difficult to believe that orthodox medicine doesn't accept the obvious fact that there is *no* degenerative disease which doesn't ultimately involve nutrition—if only at the cellular level. Let me offer you a small, true history, involving another disorder, to help you to realize the resistance of the establishment to innovative ideas. At Albert Einstein School of Medicine, a pair of identical twins were diagnosed as being autistic. At intervals, the neurology department asked the mother to bring the twins back, as an exhibit of the genetic factor in this dreadful disorder. With the hope that she might find help for the children, who had shown no response to drugs, she consulted a medical nutritionist, who undertook a study of the boys for nutritional deficiencies and for allergies that might be adversely affecting brain function. Some deficiencies were identified, almost identical in the twins; some cerebral allergies, a few quite severe, were found. Their diets were corrected, and the offending foods removed. A few months later, the Albert Einstein neurologist called the mother, asking her again to exhibit the twins at a neurological conference. She agreed, as she always had, but she told the physician that he should know that the twins were now well on their way to normalcy—playing with each other and with other children, receiving and giving affection, and communicating in speech with their teachers and parents. She told the neurologist how these gains had been achieved, and his comment was a classic example of the tunnel vision of the orthodoxy. "You can't do that," he protested. "The treatment would have to be doubleblind!" He was saying that the twins really might have responded to the power of suggestion, to a placebo effect. Which was fascinating, considering that autistic children, in the very nature of the strange disorder, live in another world, and don't respond to *anything*.

Had the problem been arthritis, and the recovery achieved with doses of B Vitamins or the no-nightshade diet, there might have been another explanation for the response: "There are spontaneous remissions in arthritis, and when they occur, the patient will, of course, give the credit to whatever treatment, however valueless, was being used at the time." This would be offered, of course, as an alternative to the power of suggestion. Oddly, science finds it necessary to guard against the possibility that faith, rather than medication, is responsible for the patient's recovery—but regards faith healers as quacks.

The laws of probability predict a "normal curve" for adequacy of diet in any large group of healthy people—meaning that their nutrition will range from atrocious to superb, with a large group falling in the middle. This is not to say that they couldn't eat more nutritiously, and be healthier. After all, an American's definition of good health includes premenstrual tension, indigestion, allergies, heartburn, constipation, flatulence, dandruff, fatigability, colds, sore throats, virus infections, and poor eyesight. Those same laws of probability apply to the diets of arthritics, and can't be repealed by the Arthritis Foundation. Among sufferers with arthritic diseases, you will find a higher than "normal" percentage of the inadequately nourished. And when you correct their diets, many of them will feel better, many will suffer less disability and pain, and some will respond with a gratifying recovery from their disease. Even in the non-responders, better nutrition will promote heightened response to medication, mitigation of side reactions, and accelerated healing after surgery.

But correction of poor diets is not the sole weapon of the medical nutritionist. Nutrient needs may skyrocket in sick people, and when needed high doses of these factors are provided, the response may surpass by far that achieved with drugs; moreover, without side reactions. (The orthodoxy in rheumatology likes to forget that Dr. Tom Spies, honored by the AMA for his pioneering research in clinical nutrition, routinely found vitamin therapy helpful in controlling the lesser pains of arthritis.)

All this is the application of positive nutrition in the treatment of this group of degenerative diseases. There is also negative nutrition—removing from the diet those foods to which the patient is sensitive, allergic, or intolerant. By deletion of offending foods from the diet, both osteoàrthritics and rheumatoid arthritics have been significantly helped—but the arthritis establishment has a blind spot for that kind of treatment, too. Even their initial premise is in error, when they claim that poor nutrition doesn't cause arthritis. More than fifty years ago, a clinician investigated two groups of hospitalized patients. The first were essentially healthy, having been hospitalized for recovery from accidents. The second had degenerative diseases—arthritis, diabetes, cardiovascular disorders, and the like. The only significant difference he could find in the backgrounds of the two groups was in their diet histories. The healthy group had eaten sensibly; the sick had a long history of poor diet.

As you will not learn about Dr. Tom Spies' use of vitamin therapy in arthritis when you read Arthritis Foundation literature, so will you remain ignorant of the lifelong research of William Kaufman, M.D., who achieved such a reputation for helping arthritics with nutritional therapies that a letter addressed to "The Arthritis Doctor, Bridgeport, Connecticut," promptly reached him. From the orthodox literature, you will never discover that Dr. John Ellis has used a simple therapy of Vitamin B6 and potassium to bring thousands of arthritis victims back to social and vocational functioning. In the Foundation literature, which persists in viewing osteoarthritis as a "wear and tear" (and thereby, inevitable) disease, you will not find a single word about the clinical research of Esther Tuttle, M.D., who successfully treated that type of arthritis as an error of the body, and benefited her patients thereby. And if you hear about the "no nightshade!" diet of Dr. Norman F. Childers, it will be in the form of a warning that Childers' statements, backed by a decade of research with thousands of arthritics, are "at best, premature; at worst, false." The Foundation's judgment, unforgivably, is an opinion based on no research at all, and the criticism itself is at best premature and at worst, false. And it *is* false.

Among the hundreds of radio stations which have aired my nutrition broadcasts, there is KFAC, in Los Angeles, on which I first publicized the no-nightshade diet for arthritis. Several months after that brief program, a listener wrote to tell me that his wife was severely arthritic, and slavishly subservient to the advice of the "big doctors" whose words of wisdom had not helped her at all, but remained her commandments, nonetheless. When he told her about my broadcast on the nightshades and their role in causing or aggravating arthritis, she repeatedly demurred with: "If this is true, why don't my doctors know it? Why wouldn't the government have told us about it?" She finally surrendered, because he refused to, and dropped from her diet the considerable amount of nightshade plants she had been eating. Her recovery from totally crippling arthritis and unbearable pain was so rapid (which it often isn't) and so complete that these simple dietary restrictions had literally converted her from an invalid into a nearly normal person. The husband's reactions were unexpected. "I think we ought to sue the government," he wrote, in indignation, undoubtedly remembering the months of needless suffering. "If these common foods can cause arthritis—even in just a few people—they must know it. Are they keeping quiet because they're protecting the agricultural industry?" I doubted that, and on the air, said so. More likely it was, I conjectured, that the government shared with most physicians and with the arthritis orthodoxy ignorance of—or rejection of—the dangers of nightshade plants to those susceptible to their toxicities.

As you will learn from this text, there is a co- and counterplay between nutrients and hormones, with the result that a deficiency of one may be displayed only as an imbalance of the other. That translates into the possibility of stimulating internal production of hormones, when it has been inadequate, rather than upsetting the glandular orchestra by introducing "soloists" on prescription. It is a possibility recognized only by the avant-garde in nutrition, though the German literature speculated upon it nearly fifty years ago. The following note, written by a physician, illustrates the application of the principle:

> Dear Doctor Fredericks:
> If I were a religious man, I should say God Bless You. Not being religious, I shall merely send my thanks—for last night I walked upstairs, using both good legs like an adult. Prior to this, I had dragged one leg and ascended with the other, because my arthritic knee gave me so much pain.
> When I heard your lecture on the support which can be given the adrenal gland by PABA, pantothenic acid, etc., I decided it would be a lot cheaper to manufacture my own cortisone than to buy it at a drugstore—not to mention the side reactions which accompany the drug. I decided to change my diet, emphasizing the foods you described as being rich in these factors, rather than using doses of the concentrated vitamins. The result was

my dramatic walk upstairs last night. It took about three months to arrive at my recovery.

Had he used the concentrated vitamins, he would undoubtedly have responded faster. Dr. Spies remarked that therapeutic nutrition must be concentrated, continuous, and consistent. But had he used the vitamin concentrates, he would, by Arthritis Foundation definition, have been a victim of Gullible's travels, and his recovery, in any event, a tribute to the power of suggestion.

What I've written is really a complaint against the cultural lag, for which medicine is notorious: the gap between a finding and its application to preventing or alleviating the suffering of humanity. To shortening that lag, I've dedicated some forty years as a professional educator in nutrition, and to that purpose, in arthritic diseases, this book is dedicated.

CARLTON FREDERICKS, PH.D., F.I.A.P.M.

1

The Biggest Deficit in Arthritis Treatment—*You*

Among the omissions in orthodox treatments for arthritis, the most significant and overlooked is *your* failure to take responsibility for your sickness and for your recovery. You must begin to take charge of your own body. Otherwise you wind up with docile swallowing of an unending series of pills prescribed by a series of physicians, with the ultimate benefits largely shared by the druggist, the pharmaceutical manufacturer, and the medical profession.

Only when the patient himself begins to participate in seeking and exploring all the possible roads to help and recovery will treatment be effective, rather than a masking of symptoms. In that sense, then, this book is a kind of trip ticket, like those provided by the automobile clubs. It is you who must choose the routes and destination. If these lead only to your surrender to medical dogma, confining you to the operating room, the physiotherapy department, and the pharmacy, don't be astonished if the treatments fail, producing benefits which are only transient and, in any case, are addressed to the symptoms rather than the underlying disease process. To put it bluntly: dividends in improved health don't rain on those who blindly worship at the shrine of medical dogma, contemplating their navels or their stiff and painful joints.

In what I've just said, there is no blame for the layman, lost in a medical world he never made, but it contains an explicit admonition: if you don't take charge of your own body, if you abdicate that responsibility, you must live with the consequences. A perfect example of what I'm saying occurs when the arthritis patient knows that he has a few allergies, or that he comes from a strongly allergic family. The process that caused asthma in your father or hay fever in your brother may in you be responsible for causing, or at least aggravating, your arthritis. Yet tests for allergy are certainly rare in rheumatological practice, in my experience, though the competent medical journals thirty-one years ago reported recovery in arthritics whose allergies were identified, and the offending foods removed from their diets. Even when allergy testing is performed, by methods which have gone unchanged for some fifty years, there is still a loophole, for the older techniques are inaccurate, yielding false negatives and false positives. Yet the allergies *can* be identified by newer methods—some of which can be used at home. None of this will happen if your share of the treatment consists of popping pills and promptly paying your doctor's bills.

If you're overweight, you certainly know it—unless you are still sticking to the old story that you're "big-boned." Fat, though, is more than an unsightly blanket. It is a monument to an ongoing and poor diet. Fat is far from inert; it actually manufactures at least one hormone, potent enough to cause infertility in women and capable of disturbing the glandular equilibrium which is essential to the "wisdom of the body." There's an excellent chance, then, that merely reducing to normal weight will improve your arthritis, even if it does nothing more than to relieve your aching joints of the extra burden.

Physiotherapy isn't the only kind of physical medicine which may help an arthritic. You may lose a possible opportunity for improvement if you don't explore the benefits of manipulative medicine—osteopathy—or chiropractic. I'm aware that many physicians consider chiropractic to be less than a science. I'm also acquainted with physicians who for their own aches and pains go to chiropractors. In England, the medical men have formed a society of manipulative medicine, on the ancient premise that, failing to lick them, you'd better join them. The question is: how far have you gone in exploring the possible benefits of such alternative or adjunct treatments?

There's another possible cause for your arthritic troubles that is never explored in standard treatment. We know that removing four popular American foods from the diet may be followed by dramatic improvement or total cure of your bursitis, tendonitis, myositis, or arthritis. (I'll explain that, in just a minute.)

One of the theoretical explanations of the cause of rheumatoid arthritis postulates a disturbance of the immune system—the mechanism in the body which guards against foreign protein, such as bacteria, viruses, and cancer. The hypothesis has it that in arthritis of this type, the immune system has gone astray, is failing to recognize normal tissue as being normal, and is reacting by attacking it. The quest based on that premise is, of course, for drugs that will make the immune system behave. So again we see the arthritis specialists blind to two factors which potently affect the immune system: nutrition and the emotions. Since the immune factors in the blood are proteins, their basic materials obviously come from the diet. One would expect a hunt for methods of controlling the diet to normalize the immune system, rather than a search for new and potent drugs—which always turn out to have side reactions.

As for the influence of the emotions on the immune system, even the highly trained physician is still unaware that this system bottoms when emotional stress rises to the point of dis-stress. It isn't coincidence that serious (and, frequently, lethal) attacks of cancer or heart disease follow periods of great emotional pressure, like the loss of a loved one. Which, of course, doesn't explain the absence of a good psychotherapist from the medical team dealing with a type of arthritis where the immune system has been compromised.

To take advantage of any of these possibilities, you'll begin by assuming some of the responsibility for the care of your body. You'll follow that by parting with a few misconceptions, erroneous but popular. One of these is voiced in the tired phrase: "Of course I have arthritis—I'm getting old." That philosophy has no relationship to reality. Time and the calendar are concepts of duration, and concepts don't cause arthritis. Time isn't toxic. Aren't there people older than you who have no arthritis problem, and thousands of children crippled with the disease?

The concept of aging as an excuse for a degenerative disease is based on correlation: aging and these disorders go hand in arthritic hand. But correlation never proves causation, though it may imply it. You can't conclude that umbrellas cause rain by demonstrating that rain always accompanies raised umbrellas. Linked with the aging theory is another one, usually invoked to explain osteoarthritis: it's a wear-and-tear disease, which, of course, combines stress with a long period of years to bring it on. But then, why does it hit only one knee in some people? Did the other one escape wear and tear? As a Vitamin B Complex deficiency may cause a sore at only one side of the mouth, so may a metabolic derangement choose at random the joints it will attack, and in any case, poor nutrition may cause the metabolic storm while weakening the structures of tissue and bone.

What you have read is the prologue to a searching look at an effective treatment for many cases of arthritis—rejected *without testing* by the establishment in the field, and yet a rewarding and harmless treatment which has been used successfully by thousands of sufferers. This, the newest and simplest and more startling treatment can be remembered by remembering this acronym:

Avoid the PPET foods.

The acronym stands for:

Potato (white)	*Eggplant*
Peppers	*Tomato*

These foods contain a toxic principle—so much of it that the amount in a human being's yearly intake of potatoes, administered to a horse, would kill it quickly. There are arthritics, of course, who don't owe their sickness to these foods, which are all of the nightshade family; but in those who are sensitive to this toxin, arthritis and other diseases, such as diverticulosis, myasthenia gravis, and depression, can be the prices for regular indulgence. From the results reported by thousands of arthritics who have used the no-nightshade diet, it appears that about seven in every ten arthritics are intolerant of them. The range goes from relative insensitivity to mild intolerance, and a large group is so sensitive that eating even a small amount of a nightshade plant brings a prompt flare-up of tenderness, pain, and stiffness of the joints.

This translates into the simplest arthritis treatment ever discovered: you simply stop eating nightshade foods. (It isn't easy to escape them, because they are ingredients in many recipes, but we'll point out those which are suspect.) If you turn out to be insensitive to these foods, you'll have dropped some favorite dishes for a few months, with no nutritional penalty—no food is unique, and others can be substituted. And if you turn out to be on the right track, all you'll lose is pain, though to what degree, no one can foretell. The diet provides grateful relief for some patients, but for others it has literally let them escape from canes and walkers.

What I'm about to say rests on two assumptions:
1. You are startled by the thought that peppers, potatoes, tomatoes, and eggplant can have caused your troubles.
2. You are going to ask your physician to read this chapter, and he will share your skepticism.

For those good reasons, let me trace for you the historical background of the nightshade plants in animal and human nutrition, in the course of which you will discover that they've been regarded as troublemakers for many centuries. Long ago, the potato was regarded with such suspicion that an English society was formed for the specific purpose of discouraging human use of the food. The tomato was a target for skepticism, too, and originally was called the "love apple" in the mistaken belief that it is an aphrodisiac. It was also called the "cancer apple," considered poisonous and productive of disease, and was and still is avoided by some Europeans. (As I write these lines, I am thinking of one of my ancestors, who, arriving here from Europe and finding the tomato on sale on pushcarts, bought and consumed one —while sitting down, for he confidently expected to be poisoned.) This was not a superstition seated in pure ignorance, for both the vines and the suckers of the tomato have been long known to be poisonous to livestock. In fact, the scientist who pioneered in evolving the no-nightshade diet for arthritis, Dr. Norman F. Childers, Blake Professor of Horticulture at Rutgers University, told me that cattle graze on wild nightshades with reluctance, and suffer from arthritic joints when they do. That was one of the clues which led him to study the possible role of these foods in human arthritis.

As the tomato was known as the "cancer apple," so was the eggplant known as the "apple of insanity," reflecting the Mediterranean belief that a month's consumption of eggplant would cause psychosis. In a time-honored method of preparation of eggplant for human meals, there may be a reflection of this ancient belief, for the housewife peels the eggplant, slices it, and salts it—to draw out the juice of insanity? Interestingly, the chemical blamed for worsening arthritis, if not for causing insanity, is concentrated in the skin area of the vegetable. (The belief about insanity may not be as wild as it seems, for the nightshade chemical which is the mischief maker for arthritics interferes with a neurotransmitter essential to brain function.)

The garden pepper is a whole family, including all the hot peppers, excluding black pepper, which would involve the tabasco pepper, and the cherry, red cluster, bell, sweet, green, pimiento, chili, long, and red peppers. Paprika, widely used in this country, is a particularly disturbing pepper for sensitive arthritics, and chili peppers—of the kind used in chili con carne—are also taboo.

The arthritic isn't a sufferer with an infrequent disease; his forlorn company runs into the millions, and the spectrum of the penalties ranges all the way from back pain—which brings nearly 20 million people to physicians and other practitioners yearly, disabling some 7 million of them—to complete crippling. A few pages ago, I told you that correlation doesn't prove cause and effect, but there is some impressive evidence. For example:

In recent years, anyone studying American dietary habits would conclude that we had decided to go on a nightshade binge. Solanine, the mischief-maker in the nightshades, is concentrated in the skins of potatoes, though present, of course, in the entire pulp, and we have discarded the traditional boiled potato with the skin removed and, seeking additional fiber in the diet, have substituted the baked potato, eaten with the skin. We have increased our intake of nightshades and solanine by using ketchup on everything but ice cream, and managed to combine two sources of solanine by drowning our French fries in ketchup. Potato chips sell in enormous volume, and are a special hazard for the solanine-sensitive arthritic, for the conversion of potatoes into chips greatly increases the surfaces exposed to light, which raises the solanine content. One need not be a nutritionist to recognize that we are nearly gorging ourselves with foods rich in tomato and peppers, such as pizza and pasta, added to increasing intake of tomato juice and of salads with tomatoes and peppers.

Conversely, countries where the nightshades are rarely consumed don't face in arthritis statistics the growing problem that we do here. A study of blacks from northern countries of Africa who were introduced to the nightshades when they came to take jobs in the Cape Town area show that some 3 percent of them develop arthritis. This, of course, raises the obvious question: why aren't Italians suffering from a 70 percent incidence of arthritis? Perhaps genetically based tolerance is the explanation; perhaps the high-nightshade diet, over the centuries, makes nonsurvivors of the highly sensitive. It is fascinating to learn that at least one Chines physician, trained in the United States, corrected his diet by going back to the Chinese diet, free of nightshades, and cured his own arthritis, leading him to set up similar menus for his arthritic patients.

Livestock that have grazed on nightshade weeds are often found kneeling, which is mute evidence of the soreness of their joints. Ordinarily, they won't eat these plants, unless they're concealed in their ordinary fodder. One can understand why livestock breeders make a special effort to remove the nightshade weeds from their pastures.

You will remember that I told you, earlier, that science has an allergy to "anecdotal evidence," regarding as valueless any observations that are made without eliminating the power of suggestion. I reject faith healing as an explanation of all the improvements patients with arthritis have enjoyed when persuaded to stop eating the nightshades. In that position, I am fortified by what happens when these responders, sometimes inadvertently, sometimes as a knowing sin, go back to eating nightshades. They usually pay a price, and sometimes a bitter one, in a flare-up of pain, stiffness, and muscular spasms after a few slices of tomato, a bit of potato salad, or a cup of cheap yogurt which has been "stiffened" with potato starch. To Dr. Childers, this suggests that the body defends itself, as best it can, when the nightshade intake is both high and regular, but loses its defences when these plants are eaten infrequently.

This closely parallels observations by allergists, who find

that patients often can't tolerate even a small amount of an offending food after they've stopped consuming the large quantities they ate regularly before they knew they were allergic. Significantly, Dr. Childers also remarks that arthritics who go back to eating baked potatoes, for instance, will observe that the food makes them sleepy. In people with addictive allergies, which are explained in chapter 3, this is a frequent observation. I don't believe that nightshade sensitivity is allergy; it's more likely toxicity, but the two reactions could be simultaneous. Certainly there are some curious parallels in them. For instance, consider the following list of symptoms:

Muscle cramps
Muscle spasms
Muscle tremor or jerking
Muscle stiffness
Muscle weakness
Aching of joints
Stiffness of joints
Swelling of joints
Myositis (inflammation of muscles)
Arthritis (inflammation of joints)

I didn't show that list to Dr. Childers, but if I had, he would have recognized it as a list of the symptoms which disappeared or improved in people with arthritis who learned to avoid the nightshade foods. Actually, the list comes from allergists. These are the symptoms elicited when some people are challenged with foods to which they are allergic. It may not appear to you to make any difference whether the pain and stiffness originate with intolerance to nightshades or with allergy. It does, and it invites research. If it is intolerance, the no-nightshade diet is the best resource. If it is allergy, other aids can be added—again, explained in chapter 3.

Over the years in which I've known Dr. Childers, he has

been kind in sending me copies of some of the reports he daily receives from the large group of arthritics who have been testing the no-nightshade diet. Let me note, before I quote from a few of them, that several of these favorable reports came from experts in horticulture—Childers' own field—who originally fought this concept with fang and claw, to the point where a society in that field actually made an effort to deny him the right to read a paper on his research. The resistance is understandable. It is proverbial that medicine has always delayed its acceptance of innovative ideas. But in horticulture, it wouldn't merely be apathy to a new concept. It would be a life-and-death struggle because Dr. Childers' work challenges the business of truck farmers, agribusiness, university departments subsidized by these industries, and government agencies slavishly subservient to the economic welfare of farmers. So the resistance is understandable, even if scientifically it is unforgivable.

The letters you are about to read are a minute percentage of the reports which Dr. Childers has received from those who have used the no-nightshade diet for arthritis; and they don't represent spontaneous comments. When the horticulturist realized that eliminating nightshades from his diet had freed him of arthritic pain and stiffness, matters took the course they always do: a few of his friends and colleagues decided to try the diet. Being a scientist, Dr. Childers wanted to organize a trial which would have meaning, and therefore he brought his findings to the attention of the public, and requested cooperation from interested arthritics. So there came into being a small army of "cooperators" running into the thousands. Each received a questionnaire, the answers to which permitted a survey of the effects of the diet. The questionnaire follows—both for your information, and because those arthritics who report on their experience with the diet, by answering these queries, will be helping to speed the day when the authorities in that field will be compelled to mount a scientific investigation of the no-nightshade treatment of this prevalent disease.

Arthritis: Don't Learn to Live with It

Survey   *No-nightshades Diet*   *Date*_____

We shall appreciate very much your help in evaluation. Please complete the questions below, and return immediately.

Name _____

State _____

Date _____

Are you on the diet? _____

If so, indicate: □ Rigidly
                   □ Somewhat
                   □ Discarded it because of negative results

Using medication now?____Previously? _____

Taking vitamins? _____

Smoking?* _____

List the problems which made you try the diet: _____

_____

_____

_____

Are you continuing the diet? _____

*Tobacco is also a nightshade

Should you decide to copy and answer the questions, after experience with the diet, your report should be sent to Dr. Norman F. Childers, Blake Professor of Horticulture, Cook College, Rutgers University, New Brunswick, N.J. 08903.

Both in the form of brief responses to the questions, and in lengthy letters, back to the pioneering horticulturist came thousands of reports on the experience of arthritics with the diet. Apropos of the last question, it is interesting to note, however variously stated, that many of the "cooperators" indicate they are *afraid* to stop the diet, for fear of losing the benefits they derived.

The problems, noted a worker with the Lupus Foundation, "included the left ankle, right ankle, under the knee, the hip. The hip would seem to catch, and I had trouble bending my right leg to tie my shoe. I have followed the diet for four months, and have been free of pain for the last month." The report is signed with the arthritic's name, preceded by two terse notations: "I am continuing the diet—afraid to stop. Thanks."

A letter with a much more detailed report came from a fellow worker in the field of horticulture, who told Dr. Childers:

> I hated passenger cars because my back hurt so much. Getting out of bed in the morning was work. A thorough examination revealed no disc problem whatsoever. I was told I had "a little arthritis" in the lower spine; nothing could be done about it. Take aspirin when the pain gets bad.
>
> Daily living was a chore. I was now in such shape I was contemplating early retirement, moving to a dry climate which might help. Then pure chance put me in the same seat section with you on the flight to Cleveland. The bag of peanuts offered by the stewardess, with paprika labeled on the bag, changed my whole life, for that brought up the subject. I began avoiding the nightshades immediately, perhaps somewhat out of desperation, but also with the attitude of having nothing really whatever to lose, and a great deal to gain. I don't think I really believed it would do anything for my back, but I was most anxious to try.
>
> [Note: the chance meeting on the airplane was in March.] I responded before March was out. I woke up one morning vaguely aware that I had not awakened to turn my body over with the long familiar routine of manipulation of the elbows to minimize the pain in the back. A night or two later it happened again. Sure enough, I had gone to sleep on one side, awakened on

the other side! That had not happened in more than three years. That gets attention! Now I observed closely, but kept the business low key all the way. By early April I was sleeping through the night without waking up to turn myself over. But I still had pain turning over *before* I went to sleep. So really it was no big deal. However, it turned out to be the beginning of a steady progression to a normal life. Painless sleep, easier driving of cars, a bit of weeding this spring and summer without problems then or later. Then in June, I arrived. I got out of bed that morning and strode to the picture window of our bedroom to view all my backyard plants —a routine of 21 years since we moved into that bedroom. But *this* morning I had gotten out of bed and strode to the window like any normal person! For the first time I had gotten up and walked away without standing still to get straightened up, or simply wait for that first back pain of the day. It *always* began then. And so for me, June 13 was the day.

This horticulturist yielded to the human tendency to try a favorite forbidden food. His wife prepared potato salad, and he indulged, half motivated by the desire to test the effect of leaving the diet. His departure from it was limited, he notes, but for two mornings he had the old back pains when he got out of bed. Mild, he notes, but unmistakable. His conclusion was inescapable—in his own words, "Clearly, I am one who was going to hell fast with the Solanaceae (nightshades) and didn't know it."

Addressed to me from one of my radio listeners who acted on a broadcast on the nightshades in arthritis, came this note:

> I was going through the trauma of worrying about my family, job, a son going to a university, bills, etc., not to mention the fear that I might become crippled from osteoarthritis. I'm sure you have seen people in

this state of anxiety. To come quickly to the point, I grasped at the idea of eliminating the nightshades from my diet because on reflection I realized that I had been eating those foods all summer and into the fall and winter. In just 2 weeks time the pain disappeared from both heels and from other parts of my feet that had started to become affected. (I could jump for joy when I think of that!)

Many of those who benefit by nuturitional treatment become evangelists—and discover that the way of the educator is hard. This correspondent sorrowfully closes with: "I have told people of my experience, hoping I could help them or someone they love from going through the pain and agony of arthritis, only to have them scoff at the idea or politely laugh it off."

Sometimes the pain blamed on an injury or a virus may be initiated, instead, by a nightshade sensitivity, or at least aggravated by it. So finds a "cooperator" who told Dr. Childers:

Fortunately for me, I read about your theory of how the nightshade plants affect our bodies. It seemed odd enough to be logical.

After living with an aggravated case of viral tendonitis since 1945, and arthritis of the back and neck caused by two auto accidents, I decided to try your no-nightshades diet. Af first I eliminated the foods that were the most obvious except when my desires overcame my common sense. In time I have learned to adhere strictly to the diet. After much experimenting, I have found that I have reactions to even the minutest amounts of the nightshades. It just isn't worth it to eat any.

No more aspirins, Valium, Motrin or Clinoril for me. Adhering to the diet of absolutely no nightshades is all it takes. Thanks for helping me.

The 70 percent success record with the no-nightshade diet tends to obscure the fact that some of the failures accrue from factors which interfere with complete avoidance of these foods. I noted earlier that there is enough potato starch in some cheap brands of yogurt, used as a thickener to give the product "body," to cause arthritis pains to flare in the solanine-susceptible. Herb teas may contain hot peppers. Many prepared dishes, often consumed by the elderly, contain white potato and tomato, which demands careful reading of labels; and the small print in which ingredients are listed may prove trying to aged eyes. Incidentally, sensitivity to the nightshades is certainly not confined to adults. One woman reported that her baby cried all day when she nursed him, after having eaten tomato the previous day.

You've now read reports from patients with arthritis and tendonitis. Among the varieties of arthritic disorders, there is one which, as a nutritionist, I should not have expected to be responsive to the no-nightshade regime. That is gout, and I was wrong. Writes a sufferer:

I have suffered from arthritis attacks for about ten years. The attacks became progressively more painful and disabling. Pain would be felt around the joints but not within them. The thighs would be affected after sitting for some time. Areas around some joints (ankles, knees, fingers, wrists) would become swollen and pain to the touch.

Medically diagnosed on two occasions as having a "gouty" disposition resulting from excessive uric acid level. No restrictions on consumption of nightshades . . . . Allopurinol was prescribed . . . this seemed to help but attacks would still occur from time to time.

Last summer, while on the drug, I experienced my worst attack and became a candidate for a wheel chair. Experienced pain around left hip, left knee, and right ankle simultaneously.

After reading an article (on the no-nightshade diet), I decided to try eliminating the nightshades from my diet. At the time, I was consuming tomatoes several times a day, and baked potatoes daily—ingesting their jackets as well. After eliminating the nightshades, improvement was noted in about three days. After about 1½ weeks, I was almost back to normal; however pain in shoulders persisted after a night's sleep and was the last to disappear.

At his time, about six months after eliminating the nightshades, I am virtually pain free and more physically active than I've been for about 10 years. I haven't taken any medication for about two months. Feel great!

A registered nurse learned two important lessons from her experience with the diet. The first was the quick penalty for slipping from grace. She wrote:

I'm happy to tell you that I'm without pain most of the time. The little pain I do have is slight in comparison with the way I was more than a year ago. I follow the diet strictly, but sometimes someone will slip paprika or such in some food when I eat out, and I know it the next day, but usually this pain is slight and goes away a day or two later.

The second lesson came as a shock to a health professional. She encountered the same insensate resistance which Dr. Childers faced from the arthritis orthodoxy. She comments:

I have tried to pass along my knowledge, but have found that no one is interested. A case in point . . . our staff orthopedist at the VA hospital is in a great deal of back (lower) pain and wears a back brace, etc., has had surgery, to no avail. I carefully mentioned the elimination of nightshades from his diet, and he read the book, but still says he couldn't possibly give up tomatoes or potatoes from his diet. I find it hard to believe that an educated person would not even try such a simple procedure. How can I expect my uneducated patients to try to rid themselves of pain, if this highly educated doctor will not try? Don't you get discouraged? It does work for me, and I am thankful for your research, and I wouldn't dare to cheat on the diet as I know I would pay dearly with much pain for about three weeks.

Not all results are dramatic, nor are all responses quick. In the sixth month of the no-nightshades diet, a correspondent remarks that his pains have lessened, but not disappeared. He isn't discouraged, realizing that the recovery, if it does eventuate, may take two years when the problem is long standing. His other notes are positive:

1. My stamina has increased quite a bit.
2. I have become able to do yard work, painting, and many other tasks that were almost impossible before.
3. The swelling in my hands etc., is completely gone.
4. I sleep from 10 p.m. to 6 a.m. nearly every day.

Sometimes the dividends from the diet are small, but very much appreciated nonetheless. A woman who endured treatments with gold salts, anti-inflammation drugs, aspirin, penicillamine, etc., wound up with her stomach "awash with ulceration." No longer able to tolerate medication, except a steroid hormone, she went on disability. We pick up her story there:

Since then I met a rheumatologist who treated arthritis with antibiotics; I started on his regime, having several bouts of ulcer trouble, and then read your article [on the no-nightshade diet]. Peppers never did agree with me nor too many tomatoes; eggplant I never ate much of. But I have always been a meat and potato eater since childhood, and thought potatoes were a healthy food. I decided to give your potato taboo a try for a month, and substituted rice, noodles, sweet potatoes, and bread filling for potatoes. To my surprise, my medicine is staying down better and my tummy is behaving more normally. This was within a few weeks of starting the non-potato diet. Keep up your good work.

A letter about a response in spinal arthritis illustrates the manner in which nightshades are unknowingly retained in the diet. A professional man's wife wrote:

Since reading the article, I have not eaten potatoes or tomatoes. That was in September. By December, sooner than I expected, I noticed a great relief from my problem, which is spinal arthritis. I have also lost much of the discomfort of indigestion with which I had lived for a long time. I hoped that these changes were due to the diet, because then I would know the specific cause of the improvement, and could continue.

Some time in January, the pain in my back and ache and pain in my legs was increasing unaccountably. After a short time, looking for the magazine article which I read originally, I found another article about your research, and read that green peppers are also of the nightshade family. I had for a while been eating peppers excessively. Needless to say, your research has created a great change in my life and outlook. I am very grateful.

There are numerous publications aimed at the elderly, and questions about arthritis are often directed to their editors. When the answers follow the "party line" of the arthritis orthodoxy, those who have benefited by the no-nightshade diet are, understandably, upset. In response to an attack on the diet in such a magazine, a subscriber wrote:

I was very disappointed to read the answer to the first question in your September issue. I have had osteoarthritis for five years and have not been without pain. I had changed my lifestyle to "easing around" to avoid aggravating the condition. Two months ago, I started the [no-nightshade] diet, and I have been free of arthritic pain since then. I have gone from taking anti-inflammatory drugs and 15 aspirin per day, on my doctor's recommendation, to 4 aspirin per day. I have also been able to resume normal physical activity without pain. My hands aren't stiff every morning, any more. My whole life has been changed because of this diet, and your article calls it "worthless remedy" and "no value whatsoever." I am appalled. Would it have been wrong to suggest to the person who was inquiring that it certainly wouldn't hurt to cut these [nightshade] foods out of their diets on a trial basis? You could still have a "well balanced diet of varied nourishing foods" without using the nightshades. You could still follow your doctor's orders while trying this diet. I did.

If you knew of this diet, developed by Dr. Norman F. Childers, and still answered as you did, SHAME ON YOU. If you were unaware of his work, I suggest that you write to him at Rutgers University. He has records to prove that people have been helped by this diet.

The magazine took its editorial philosophy from statements of the Arthritis Foundation, who should have received the scolding directly—which their Atlanta chapter did, for in response to the same article, an arthritic wrote:

I was so angry when I read the article. Until December 18, 1978 I would have accepted all your conclusions. On that important date of my life I was fortunate to read about Dr. Childers' "no-nightshades diet." Having suffered with painful arthritis for twenty-five years, I was feeling worse each year. I've been on his diet for ten months, and feel better and better as time goes by. You'll never convince me that omitting nightshades from my diet has not accomplished this. Since you are supported by public donations, I believe that you must start to give publicity for people to try this diet. What have they to lose but pain? What will you lose? Nothing. But [you will gain] gratitude from a suffering public. Remember Sister Kenny and the abuse she suffered from organized medicine? . . . I do hope to see a constructive attitude from your organization.

A retired army officer, 71 years old, suffering with arthritis for 20 years, writes a report which indicates that neither age nor duration of the problem are necessarily bars to response. In terse language, he remarks:

Nov., 1978, walking very painful, difficulty going up steps, every step a painful act. Went on diet in December, 1978, missing a few, such as hot pork sausage, etc. However, in July, 1979, I could walk without pain. I could even stand up and put on my trousers without sitting down. When my garden came [in], I started eating tomatoes on the 14 of July, 1979. Within six days, the pain had returned, *but bad*. I immediately quit tomatoes. It took until last week (Nov., 1979) to get back to a no pain existence. I have made arrangements to have new X-rays taken. If [in comparison with the previous ones] there is any change, I shall send you a copy. Thank you for a wonderful cure.

Dr. Childers has received many "God Bless You's," and the following report adds to that chorus:

I guess I started the no-nightshade diet in June, 1979. My one finger was badly swollen and red at the end, eventually becoming an enlarged joint such as old people get (I'm 66 now), if left alone. Well, I thought, this is one evidence I can see—let's see if it improves. It has!

And then I've discovered, as I walk the dogs lately, I seem to have *loose* joints. Sometimes really relaxed. On change of weather, the pain is not very noticeable . . . . God Bless You! and whatever source that led me to your diet. I have been fighting [arthritis] for 35 years!

Problems which originate with disturbed metabolism come ultimately to be looked upon as more or less mechanical, like the locking of arthritic joints when in the "wrong" position. They too sometimes yield to the diet, and a typical example appears in this letter from a 61-year-old:

I became aware of the diet less than a year ago. I have used potatoes, tomatoes, peppers and eggplant freely for most of my life. Tomatoes were a favorite food in the summer, and since moving to the New Mexico region I had become a fan of chili.

About two years ago I began to be seriously concerned about my increasing inability to move my body freely, especially from a stooping position to an erect posture. I had speculated to myself that in a few more years I might not be able to get out of bed. I was having trouble with my knees due to what was described by my doctor as loose cartilage, which moved about while walking, and made an almost audible sound. In the extreme bent position, my knee would lock on the obstructions. When driving a car, my right knee would begin to give me pain after a few minutes on the gas pedal.

After stopping the use of the offending plants, all of the ailments mentioned were considerably reduced, and my knee problems have virtually disappeared.

This member of Dr. Childers' "cooperator" group mentions that he has diverticulosis. It is a fairly common ailment, its cause—and cure—unknown. One theory has it that lack of fiber in the diet may be the problem, since it induces constipation, which ultimately forces the person to use undue pressure in elimination, thereby exerting tremendous force upon the colon and causing the bagging of the tissues which is the characteristic of the disease. Dr. Childers believes that sensitivity to the nightshades may also be responsible, by a totally different pathway of action, both for diverticulosis and diverticulitis, the latter involving the same disorder embellished with inflammation of the intestinal "pockets."

The skepticism of the arthritis establishment isn't shared by medical men whose minds are open. A Kent, Washington, practitioner of nutrition and holistic medicine wrote a letter to Dr. Childers, in which he offers the theory that the normalization of metabolic erros in arthritics on the no-nightshade diet actually may confirm the results which were obtained by doses of the B Complex vitamin by Dr. William Kaufman, whose nutritional therapies for the diseases are discussed in chapter 6. The chemistry he offers is persuasive, and begs for an investigation which, given the resistance of the orthodoxy to new ideas, isn't likely to be mounted by them. I am inclined again to remark that, were I a practicing rheumatologist, I'd count myself as remiss if any patient with arthritis didn't receive a trial of both the Childers diet and the Kaufman vitamin therapies.

It isn't only that the no-nightshade thesis has been rejected without examination, but the irony becomes apparent when one realizes that drugs commonly prescribed for arthritics include at least one which is *made* from a nightshade. The substance is atropine, and the drug, prescribed for digestive complaints which remind many arthritics that these disorders are *total*, not just diseases of the joints, is Lomotil. An arthritis patient writes about this:

> I began the experiment because I had nothing to lose except pain, if that were possible. I really didn't expect it to help, as doctors could give me no advice or remedy except pain-killers. Within two or three weeks [on the diet] I no longer suffered the pain in finger, wrist, and ankle joints at night. After 10 weeks of following the diet strictly, I was tempted to eat tomato-cheese pizza. Three

nights later I felt the results in knees and elbows. I then ate some potato and tomato dishes over the period of a month, and had recurrences of pain, so decided it wasn't worth eating those foods.

I no longer have heel spurs. I can now turn my head to look over a shoulder without "seeing stars" as formerly. That had bothered me for several years. Since your card pointing out Lomotil as containing a nightshade, other aches and pains have eased up. There I was, getting atropine from my colitis prescription.

I've been taking a botany course this summer at Northern Arizona University. My instructor personally knows three or four other people who have gained remarkable benefits from the "no-nightshades" diet.

The only real problem is a chronic back pain, and sometimes hips or knees aching a little, but those have bothered for many years and may improve as time goes by. My botany instructor was glad to hear I'd joined your experiment.

The botanist referred to isn't the only peer who has learned that Dr. Childers is on the right track. A world-famous researcher wrote:

Back 2 or 3 years ago, I was bothered by hip trouble. On the golf course, the pain in my right hip was often so severe that it was necessary to stop periodically and rest. Looked as if I was headed for a hospital and an artificial joint. After avoiding the nightshades there seemed to be a slight improvement but I wasn't sure and therefore said nothing. Now I am sure. No more pain. This note is therefore another piece of news of much importance to me and the means of conveying another "thank you" to you.

In radio broadcasting for forty years, I have often had the feeling that one's words are flung into the wild yonder—to fall on unhearing ears? Frequently, though, notes like this one reach my desk, from a listener who heard my radio interview with Dr. Childers:

> I want to thank Dr. Childers for helping me rid myself of the pains of arthritis. For eight months I avoided all nightshades—no pains. I continued the diet for eighteen months, and I was fine, and then, about a month ago I tried a medium size tomato, and all was fine, and then about 10 days later, pains returned in right hip and back. This was just an experiment, and you may be sure that I won't experiment any more.
>
> I suffered with arthritis pains for many years, trying spas, medications, but to no avail. For a time it helped, but not for long. When I heard about the nightshades through Dr. Fredericks, I decided I had nothing to lose but pain. I am very grateful for what you have done.

Not all orthodox physicians must plead guilty to a closed mind, as this note indicates:

> John has checked in regularly with an arthritis specialist at Hahnemann Medical School. This doctor has seen no further deterioration. In fact, the knee that had to be drained has needed no further attention. John has gotten back on his bicycle, and does four laps of a loop consisting of several long blocks. I'm less agile, and confine my activities to two long walks a day, and some riding on the bicycle we have in our T.V. room.
>
> For my part, my hands are no worse in disfigurement. I do have considerably better use of them. I prefer to take lecture notes long-hand at my conferences and meetings, and am again able to do this. In fact the quality of my longhand writing is much improved. Of no consequence to anyone but me is the fact that I can now wear some favorite rings which I thought I had put away forever.

Our physician, who is a fine human being as well as an able general practitioner, read your book with interest and an open mind, and has made inquiries from time to time.

Apologizing for the fact that a small pension and Social Security is all he has, an arthritic apologizes for not being able to contribute to the nightshade research which yielded him so many benefits. He writes:

I have followed your advice on the nightshades, and as a result my pains have left me . . . and you apologize for the price of the book???

I used to dread going to sleep at night because I would roll over on my side (either side) and the pain would wake me up. I couldn't even comb my hair unless I bent my head down so's I could reach it without raising my arm too high. My left thigh would ache until I took aspirin.

Now I'm building my own retirement home . . . handling heavy lumber, 4x8 sheets of plywood, climbing ladders, and the thousand and one things that are entailed in the building of a house. I could never have done it without your advice on the nightshades.

All the nightshades, with the exception of tobacco which I gave up about 25 years ago, were my favorite foods . . . a stew without potatoes and green bell peppers—never! Spaghetti sauce without tomatoes??? Eggplant I'd have once in a while. I don't use any of them any more except by mistake when I buy a canned food without reading the label, and I'm soon aware of it with a return of the aches. Enclosed is ten dollars to further the work. I do wish it could be more but it's all I can spare. And from the very bottom of my heart, thank you.

In a letter from a registered nurse, another common complaint of arthritics is traced to nightshade sensitivity. She reports that she appears to have two different types of arthritis —traumatic gouty arthritis, and another type which also appears at intervals but isn't helped by the medication which relieves the gouty type.

> . . . pains and stiffness in my hands became gradually more severe, until I had to use two hands to turn a door knob. When I learned about the diet, it suddenly dawned on me that my problem had started in July just as my tomatoes had come into season and I had eaten them every day. I also suddenly remembered that I had often had real gastro-intestinal distress from eating other members of the nightshade family of vegetables. Any potatoes that were not thoroughly cooked would give me violent distress. I soon learned not to eat "french fries" because they sometimes have uncooked centers. Green tomato relishes and green peppers also gave me violent intestinal pain which was not associated with gas.
>
> I am familiar with the reactions to the chemicals derived from the nightshade plants used in medical therapy, and your discovery has helped me to understand some of my food sensitivities. I have stopped eating tomatoes, potatoes, peppers and eggplant since October [her letter is written five months later] and the discomfort in my hands has now completely disappeared.

The nurse shares my mental allergy to the resistance of the orthodoxy to new ideas. She remarks:

> It appears to me that the medical profession is very reluctant to accept the theories of other professionals as it relates to clinical application. . . . I would certainly hope that some doctors would have enough interest in helping their patients that they would consider your proposal in treating suitable patients. I am sure that diet can do no harm, and that is more than I can say for almost every drug that is being used for rheumatic and arthritic

conditions. My severe reaction to even aspirin makes drug therapy almost impossible.

The reference to indigestion caused by the nightshades brings up other types of mischief created in the susceptible. A few pages back I mentioned the nursing mother whose infant cried all day after she had eaten tomatoes. Transmission of solinase in breast milk is possible—other chemicals find their way to it. A sufferer with myasthenia gravis (grave weakening of the muscles) reports complete recovery on the diet, accompanied by supplements of choline, pantothenic acid, and manganese. Since I was the first researcher to advise physicians to use those nutrients in myasthenia gravis, this report would seem to bring up the possibility that it was the nutritional supplements which helped the patient. Not so: the supplements ultimately are aimed at improving the response to the same neurotransmitter—acetylcholine—with which the solinase of the nightshade plants interferes. It is known that cattle fed the nightshades may develop diverticulosis, a disorder to which I referred earlier, and the possible role of these foods in causing human diverticulosis and diverticulitis remains to be demonstrated conclusively. Not so with their contribution to arthritis. Even though you've read just a few of the thousands of favorable reports from those who participated in the experiment, are you not convinced that any arthritic who eats significant amounts of the nightshades deserves a trial of the diet? And perhaps that adjective "significant" amounts should be less conservative, for there are those who are strikingly affected by small amounts. I mentioned earlier that the potato starch used to give body to cheap yogurt is sometimes enough to cause trouble for susceptible arthritics, and that is certainly a small amount. Dr. Childers notes that some of following hints have proved helpful to his band of experimenters:

Herb teas often contain numerous herbal ingredients, and among them may be hot pepper, paprika, or capsicum. This is the botanical name for pepper other than the black and white varieties—which are in a different family than the nightshades, and thereby unobjectionable. You must read labels.

Chocolate sometimes causes pain in the neck, feet, and hands, even though the no-nightshade diet is being meticulously followed.

Some Vitamin C pills advertised as of "natural origin" may be derived from or contain green or red pepper, which may cause trouble. Vitamin C itself—ascorbic acid—sometimes causes adverse reactions, though the natural vitamin in fruits and vegetables has been innocent. The problem here is identifying the source of the reaction, for tablets contain a number of binders, fillers, etc., to any one of which sensitivity or intolerance is possible.

Reports indicate that nightshade-reactors sometimes develop aches with frequent consumption of asparagus, beets, spinach, and rhubarb. If you find that daily use of these foods makes you react unfavorably, you can still consume them, usually, by the "four-day rotation" type of diet— in which no food is taken more than once in any four-day period. This method is often successful for those who have multiple allergies to foods, to the point where taking all the troublemakers out of the diet becomes impractical.

Troubled by inability to chew properly, because of ill-fitting dentures or uncompensated loss of teeth, some elderly people buy the strained baby foods. Reading labels is again a must, for some of these products contain white potato and tomato in sufficient quantities to touch off intolerance in the susceptible.

Cheese, particularly cheese foods and cheese spreads, but also true cheeses, may contain paprika. Since this is a particularly active troublemaker for the nightshade-sensitive, be careful about consuming products with a pinkish tint, if the label doesn't identify spices present in the food.

The earlier mention of chocolate may, in the minds of

those who realize that the stimulant in this food is related to caffeine, have raised questions about tea, coffee, and cola drinks. Some of Dr. Childers' subjects report that excessive amounts of coffee may cause a rash, and several indicate that aches in the left chest follow overindulgence. Tea may be guilty, too. No reports on cola drinks are yet available, but any nutritionist would try to persuade the healthy as well as the arthritic to avoid these concoctions of acid, concentrated sugar, and caffeine. (Among other accusations, caffeine is accused of causing cancer, deformation of the unborn young, and breast cysts in susceptible women.)

Earlier in this discussion, I mentioned the fact that in a year's intake of potatoes, a human being swallows enough solanine to kill a horse, if given in one dose. Because the following report involves this, the suspect substance in the nightshades, I'm going to ask you to read an abstract of a technical paper on this subject. It appeared in the *Quarterly Journal of Medicine*, 48 (1979), 227–43, and told the story of seventy-eight schoolboys who were made ill by eating potatoes for lunch on the second day of the fall school term. Seventeen of them were sick enough to require hospitalization, three of these being dangerously ill. The symptoms developed in seven to nineteen hours after the meal, including vomiting, diarrhea (sometimes violent), and abdominal pain, which in one child was so severe that, mistakenly, he was operated on for appendicitis. Since a feeling of depression has been reported as a reaction to nightshades—both in arthritics and nonarthritics—it is striking that these children showed a wide variety of disturbances of the nervous system, including sleepiness, outright coma, extreme restlessness, confusion, hallucinations, and visual disturbances.

The source of the trouble was an unusually high level of solinase in the potatoes, which were left over from the summer term and had probably been exposed to light, which increases the level of the toxin in the food. (For the benefit of readers with a technical background, let me note that the sick children were found to have low levels of plasma cholinesterase activity, which is a known effect of the solanidine alkaloids. The level of solanine in peeled, boiled potatoes left over from the meal was almost three times that in most whole potatoes.)

The authors of the paper speculate on the infrequency of solanine poisoning. They note that the chemical is mainly present in the peel and is soluble in water; thereby peeling and boiling would remove much of it. But they also offer the possibility that isolated cases may be overlooked, and the true frequency of excess exposure will remain unknown. They are concerned with the significance in terms of deformation of the unborn young. This book is concerned, obviously, with the greater possibility that *chronic* poisoning with solanine does occur, but isn't recognized because it's called *arthritis*.

Most housewives are aware that a green area in a white potato is somehow undesirable, and will cut it out and discard it. They are unaware that the solanine concentrated in that spot is present in the entire potato. And even those arthritics who know they are sensitive to the nightshades do not realize that common commercial practices in handling potatoes make them more dangerous. Not infrequently, potatoes are exposed to light after harvesting and again in transportation and, particularly, in the marketplace. Even in the nonsensitive, it is a good practice not to take your supply of potatoes from the top of the pile, exposed to light. As for potato chips, here the problems multiply, for the thin slices vastly expose the surface which can be exposed to light.

When an arthritic is depressed, the diagnosis is facile. Who escapes depression when threatened with a crippling and painful disease? But that melancholia may have nothing to do with the mental impact of a progressive physical disorder. It may be caused by the biochemical disturbance which causes the arthritis. To understand what I am saying, you must appreciate the fact that the psychiatrist who prescribes an anti-depression drug is making an explicit statement about the brain chemistry of the depressed patient. He is altering a neurotransmitter: one of the brain chemicals which shape our

emotional reactions, our thinking, and, indeed, our person-
alities. Among these, there is acetylcholine, a deficiency of
which has been blamed for a type of senile dementia (second
childhood). This versatile component of the chemistry of
thinking is also involved in muscle function, as my previous
reference to myasthenia gravis indicates; and the nightshades,
you must now realize, disturb acetylcholine metabolism. This
means that in those who are intolerant of the nightshades,
there may be a subgroup whose reactions are not only physical, in the form of arthritis, but mental. I am reminded here
that more than fifteen years ago, I published the observation
that lecithin—a food factor normal to the body—had a remarkable effect in reducing irritability in some people.

The relationship of the nightshades to arthritis in the susceptible is well established in the thousands who have profited by the diet. The effects of these foods in contributing to
myasthenia gravis, diverticulosis, lupus, diverticulitis, muscle
spasm—including the heart—and depression remain challenges for future investigators.

A more immediate problem is securing the cooperation of
your physician. It isn't that there is any danger in a diet which
eliminates a few common foods. The trouble comes from interaction of drugs with the diet—particularly cortisone and
gold. Dr. Childers finds that any form of cortisone, or injections of gold, will nearly always delay the response to the diet,
and he urges that medication of all kinds should be gradually
reduced—not suddenly stopped—while you are testing the
no-nightshade regime.

Another problem begins with your (understandable) dream
of an overnight cure, or at least relief. The longer the duration of the disease, and the older you are, the longer it may
take for a response. In 30 percent of the subjects, remember,
there is no benefit. But if you are in the other 70 percent—
which does give you seven chances in ten—you will never find
out, if you only toy with the diet for a month or two, then
drop it. Give it—and yourself—a chance.

2

Allergy in Arthritis— Another Stepchild

If nutrition in arthritis has been contemptuously rejected, allergy has simply been ignored, though allergic reactions may imitate, initiate, or aggravate arthritis. There is, at that, some consistency in what passes for thinking in the arthritis establishment: if food has nothing to do with arthritis, then allergy to food is even less related. Yet allergists, like nutritionists, have proved their cases, for both have helped arthritics, and the allergists have added proof: they've not only helped arthritics by removing offending foods from their diets, but they've produced fresh arthritic attacks by refeeding those foods.

With significant evidence like that tossed aside unexamined, more subtle clues are, of course, unrecognized. Example: rheumatologists at a Swedish hospital reported that they found rheumatoid arthritics improving when placed on fasts. The benefits, they noted, were temporary, for while fasting the patients had effective reduction in pain, joint swelling, and stiffness, but suffered a return of their symptoms when they resumed a full diet. The specialists offered no explanation for the ephemeral benefits, but a layman in one of my radio audiences promptly arrived at a correct interpretation. "This," he wrote to me, enclosing a copy of the Swedish report, "is what you really call missing the clue!" It was obvious to him and to me, but not to the rheumatologists, that it wasn't fasting of itself that relieved the patients' symptoms, but freedom from food to which they were allergic. Fasting, in fact, is a standard device with many allergists when they want to "wipe the slate clean" or, as they sometimes put it, completely detoxify the patient, after which foods are tested individually, and allergic reactions and their causes more easily identified.

Actually, there are allergists who strongly insist that "arthritis" is a misnomer when applied to some allergic patients, whose joint pains, stiffness, and swelling are symptoms of allergy, exactly as hives, asthma, or hay fever may be. Dr. Marshall Mandell tells the story of a patient which perfectly illustrates how allergy can trigger arthritis. He was food-testing a group of patients whose allergies caused respiratory symptoms, such as asthma. During a test for corn allergy, a woman reacted with pain in her left ankle where, she said, she had a history of arthritis as her only symptom of the disease. Dr. Mandell more accurately labeled it as an allergic reaction. In fact, in some patients whose "arthritis" is bodywide, this physician has demonstrated that the problem is bodywide allergy. Such sensitivity to food (or chemicals) may be at work in the arthritics who tell you that their aches and pains increase before a change in the weather. These living barometers aren't victims of imagination, but the sensitivity to weather changes may be aggravated by allergic reactions.

I'm sure I need not warn you that allergy isn't involved in all cases of arthritis, any more than nightshade sensitivity is —but you're entitled to the investigation, aren't you? (People totally free of allergies are *rare*. That would include arthritics.) The important point is the possibility that allergy may cause, aggravate, simulate, or be uninvolved in arthritis, but you'll never know—and you may lose an opportunity for real and lasting help—if you're not tested. Such tests are rare in the practice of the orthodox rheumatologist. Papers on the subject are vanishingly rare in the journals he reads. As a matter of fact, tests for allergy as a factor in arthritis aren't frequent in allergists' offices, nor in their medical journals. There is a small band of avant-garde medical nutritionists and bioecological allergists who do routinely make such investigations for arthritic patients, and in the Appendix, this book will guide you to their medical societies, from whom you can obtain referrals.

Years ago, I noticed that one's favorite foods often turned out to be those which caused allergy. I even suggested that allergists could dispense with testing by asking patients to stop eating the foods they liked the most and ate the most frequently. At the time, I attributed that to our tendency to become allergic to foods to which we are addicted. It never occurred to me that I had it backwards: we tend to become addicted to the foods to which we are allergic. That phenomenon is no longer a speculation. It is distinguished from other types of allergy by its name: addictive allergy. That translates as your craving for milk, for instance, possibly being based on allergy to it. That allergy can be responsible for symptoms ranging from schizophrenic behavior to ulcerative colitis—or arthritis. Let me make it clear that this is different from the nightshade reaction, which probably owes more to toxicity than to allergy.

The easiest way to explain the effects of addictive allergy is to compare it with addiction to a narcotic. It isn't only the "high" the drug addict is seeking; he is inexorably driven to the next dose because he must avoid the withdrawal symptoms—the "low." That process may be behind your craving for a food to which you are allergic. A dose of it gives you a "high"; withdrawal from it will give you a "low." The "high" is explicitly recognized in one of the tests for allergy, where the stimulation (high) from eating an allergenic food is revealed by a sharp rise in the pulse rate. All these technicalities aside, it's easily possible that you're allergic, and if you are, the odds are that the problem hasn't been explored for possible relationship to your arthritis. The absence of symptoms of addiction doesn't mean that you're not allergic, and allergy if present isn't necessarily related to your arthritis, but the question must be asked—and competently answered. As you will learn later in this chapter, that doesn't mean the usual "scratch" and "patch" tests, which long ago should have been replaced with more accurate methods, for these techniques give too many false positives and too many false negatives, and you may wind up avoiding foods that are innocent and, which is worse, continuing to eat those which are disturbing you.

The urgency of addictive allergic craving is beyond description for anyone who hasn't experienced or at least observed it, as have many medical nutritionists. One practitioner, a friend of mine, suspected a patient of addiction to chocolate, and found his supply exhausted of the chocolate syrup he used for testing. He asked the patient to go to a neighborhood bakery to buy a chocolate cookie. Instead, she purchased a three-layer chocolate cake, and managed to down it all before she returned to the doctor's office. Another practitioner tells of a hospitalized patient suffering from allergic addiction to hydrocarbons, which drove him into psychotic behavior. In the absence of supplies of glue, gasoline, and other hydrocarbons to satisfy his craving, he would sniff deeply at varnished wood doors in the hospital. The smell made him, he said, feel better. Actually, he was describing relief of withdrawal symptoms by minute "neutralizing doses," which is what he obtained by inhaling the odor of the varnish. We'll discuss that phenomenon later, but meanwhile, reflect on this: the foods you eat frequently because they make you "feel better" may similarly be masking withdrawal symptoms of the allergic reactions which can be aggravating your arthritis.

If you pause to reflect, you'll realize that you're familiar with the processes I've been describing. Who has not encountered the alcoholic who needs a morning drink—the "hair of the dog" that bit him—to mask his withdrawal symptoms, and restore the high?

The first important steps toward diagnosing possible allergy—addictive or nonaddictive—can be taken by you. Obvious clues are very likely to leap from the pages of a double-entry diary in which you list all foods, beverages, chemicals, and drugs to which you've been exposed, plus the date and time for each. In the other column, again with date and time, you list your symptoms, paying particular attention as an arthritic to swelling, pain, and stiffness in the joints. If allergy is at work, relationships will gradually come into focus. "Gradually," because pain or stiffness doesn't necessarily increase an hour (or for that matter, a day) after you eat an offending food; but if allergy is igniting your arthritis, the double-entry diary will ultimately yield important links between meals (or snacks) and symptoms. I must emphasize that the relationship won't leap out of your notes with an attention-arresting bugle call. The tomato in which you indulge after being off nightshades for months may trigger pain three days later. The corn you shouldn't have eaten may increase muscle spasm in hours, the next day, or two days later. Usually, the reaction appears fairly promptly, but people—like allergies—differ in their degree and timing of response to allergic insult.

I must again emphasize that *everything* you swallow, inhale, or contact is suspect until proved innocent. At any rate, the clues your diary may provide will not only guide you, but will be valuable to your physician too. Taking that diary to a conventional rheumatologist or, for that matter, an orthodox allergist will probably be a waste of time. Astonishingly, these specialists will grant that allergy can affect every organ and tissue in the body, but draw the line at its causing or aggravating arthritis. I regard these practitioners as hostages to the cultural lag in medicine, and propose, if you want to try to help yourself, that you not join them.

Incidentally, if you want some examples of the research ignored by both arthritis and allergy specialists, read *How to Control Your Allergies* by Robert Forman, Ph.D., published by Larchmont Books. On page 17 you'll find a list of the muscular and skeletal symptoms which have been traced to allergy. They include arthritis, joint pains, muscle cramps, muscle pains, muscle spasms, and muscular weakness. Dr. Forman supplies medical documentation for that list.

Because of the inadequacies of the scratch and patch tests for allergy, other methods have been devised which, as usual, are targets for medical controversy. These include the RAST, cytotoxic, sublingual, and Rinkel tests. Objections range from expense—which seems a little forced, since nothing is so expensive as less accurate tests—to quarrels about the principle behind a given test, or its sensitivity. Suffice it to say that these methods are all helpful in diagnosis when administered and interpreted by a competent practitioner, and they all have advantages over the older methods. In addition, there are several techniques—other than the food-symptom diary—which the layman can use as a method of identifying food, chemical, and drug sensitivities. Among these is one which, if you've never seen it used, will startle you. It is based on weakening of "indicator" muscles when you are in contact with something to which you are allergic. "Contact" may be a few drops of a solution of the food, placed under your tongue, where absorption is fast. Physicians tend to shy away from such a method, for the reason that they must rely on your subjective reactions, rather than symptoms—such as hives or reddening of the skin, in the scratch-patch methods—which they can themselves observe. The objection, it seems to me, is frivolous: if a food solution under the tongue makes you dizzy, gives you a headache, makes you feel depersonalized, or causes a flare-up of pain in an arthritic joint, your report is as meaningful as any of the external observer, however highly trained.

The point at which the orthodox physician will yield to despair comes when you are tested for allergy by holding the food in your hand. Astonishingly, in many subjects, an allergic reaction will be indicated by weakening of a muscle.

To perform this test, you need the help of an assistant. You extend one arm sideways, parallel with the floor. Your "tester," using one hand, tries the "springiness" of your arm, and you resist. It isn't a contest of strength—the tester should use about the amount of effort he'd need to lift eight or ten pounds. Now you hold the test food in the *other* hand, and repeat the test on the opposite arm. If the muscle noticeably weakens, it is strong evidence that you are allergic to— or intolerant of—that food. To avoid the power of suggestion, it is best that you not know the identities of the food which you are holding and testing. Needless to say, the specialists who perform such tests—kinesiologists—employ more than one muscle as an indicator, but one is enough for you, as an average person, to provide clues to possible allergies. Don't discount this method because you find it hard to believe that holding a food can weaken muscles elsewhere in the body. I have seen disbelieving patients proceed to eat foods which had been indicted by the kinesiological tests, with the results that their arthritic joints flared in pain, swelling, and stiffness, or they became depressed, or they developed headaches, indigestion, diarrhea, and other symptoms which can be caused by allergy. When kinesiological testing is performed by a professional, with more than one muscle used as an indicator, the tests become more sensitive thereby.

A few paragraphs ago, I mentioned a rise in the pulse rate as a symptom of allergy. This observation, originally made by his wife, was published by Dr. Arthur F. Coca, dean of allergists in America. Finding his wife's pulse at an abnormal 180 per minute, he was astonished when Mrs. Coca remarked that this was the effect when she ate something to which she was allergic. Over a period of years, Dr. Coca exhaustively tested the pulse-rate method of diagnosing allergies and found it useful for many patients. "Many" means what it indicates: there are those whose pulse doesn't reflect allergic stimulation at all. There are instances where a given food will stimulate an abnormal pulse rise at one time and not at another. This bespeaks not only a variability in pulse response to allergy, but an unpredictability in allergy itself. I know of patients who can't tolerate certain foods when they are under the "normal" stress of business, but can eat them freely when they're vacationing. In fact, I know several individuals who manage, on occasion, to be allergic to antihistamine (antiallergy) medications. The fact that the pulse rate is not an infallible test for allergy is, obviously, not an indictment.

To use Dr. Coca's method, it would be wise to read his book *The Pulse Test* (New York: ABC Books, 1959), which can still be found in paperback in some book and health stores. But I can give you an idea of how the pulse test is conducted and interpreted. This method, incidentally, really calls for keeping a diary, in order to establish links, if any, between exposure to allergens and changes in the pulse rate. The food-symptom diary described earlier would be a perfect vehicle for these added observations, which would make it even more useful.

To chart your pulse variations, you take your pulse when you awaken in the morning, before rising. You take it again just before eating. If you have good reason to suspect that you're allergic, and that this may be worsening your arthritis, eat just *one* food, so that any change in the pulse rate can definitely be traced to that food alone. Take your pulse again a half hour after eating the single food, and an hour after. If your pulse goes up more than sixteen beats at the half-hour or one-hour mark, or if it goes over 84, regardless of the amount of the rise, there is a probability that you're allergic to that food. If the pulse remains at 84 or less, or doesn't rise more than sixteen beats at the one-hour mark, you then eat another food, and repeat the testing of the pulse. If the first food is innocent, another portion of it may be taken with the second food tested, and in this way, you can track down your food allergies in a reasonably short period and without going hungry.

Dr. Coca also performed tests after full meals, recording the pulse a half hour, an hour, and an hour and a half after eating. The same criteria apply: if the pulse doesn't rise more than sixteen beats per minute, or in any case go over 84, *the entire meal can then be assumed to be innocent of causing allergic reactions—with one proviso: that meals must consist of foods you eat regularly, because the body tends to desensitize itself when there are long periods between consumption of an allergenic food. That phenomenon can, of course, lead you astray with any method of allergy testing. On the other hand, it obviously can be useful, and it *is* put to use in the four-day rotation diet, which I'll discuss shortly.

The full-meal test sounds like an easier way than the single-food method, and it is, of course—when the test is negative. But if your pulse races after a full meal, you don't know which food or foods may be responsible, and that will necessitate your returning to the single-food method to spot the mischief-maker—which, don't forget, doesn't have to be a food. You could be allergic to the cornstarch in the gravy, or the dye, Red #3, in a pudding, or to a seasoning agent.

Many laymen, in taking the pulse, count it for ten or fifteen seconds and multiply for the minute value. Coca, like most physicians, doesn't trust the accuracy of that method, preferring that you count for a full sixty seconds, using the second hand of your watch for accurate guidance.

Earlier, I referred to the four-day rotation diet, which by prolonging intervals between repeating foods in your menus, allows the body to regain its "balance," thereby bringing allergies under control. There are some qualifications for that statement:

> 1. For some individuals, four-day intervals between repeats of foods isn't long enough. Some people need five, six, or even eight days.

*A pulse which is consistently over 84 is also misleading. It may mean that the person is allergic to so many foods that the whole-meal test becomes inapplicable.

2. Some people are so exquisitely sensitive that they will remain allergic to foods even though they haven't consumed them for months. For them, no interval is long enough, and no quantity of the offending food too small to be troublesome.

Nonetheless, the rotation diet can bring priceless relief to many arthritics whose troubles are being magnified by food allergies. The emphasis on arthritis symptoms shouldn't obscure other possible dividends which can accrue from avoiding allergic reactions. A famous allergist once remarked that we don't catch colds—we eat them. Not only is the statement accurate, but it carries a pointed message for allergic arthritics, for whom any infection can increase pain and stiffness. Add to that relief from chronic indigestion, fatigue, irritability, or insomnia, and you can understand why patients are grateful to the avant-garde allergists who take the time and trouble to track down their sensitivities.

The rotation diet obviously can be used as a *test* for allergy, on the simple premise that therapeutic results point to cause. Which is to say that if your arthritis is better when you rotate foods, it argues strongly for allergy as part of your problem. This is called "therapeutic diagnosis." The physician can't logically object to it, for he uses it. A good example is the prescription of colchicine for an arthritic. If it helps, it establishes a diagnosis of gout, for this drug is specific for gout and unhelpful for other kinds of arthritis. That, too, is therapeutic diagnosis.

I don't want to pause here to give you the details of a four-day rotation diet, which requires many pages of suggested menus and lists of food families, where relationships are close enough so that allergy to one member may mean allergy to the others. You will find such information in the Appendix.

The rotation diet, the food diary, and the pulse and

kinesiological tests will give you a start. If they indicate the chance that you do in fact have an allergy problem, it will be rewarding to visit a competent physician, who can pin down the offending allergens, with your diary to supplement what he learns with tests like the RAST, Rinkel, Sublingual, and cytotoxic. But I must repeat that a "competent physician" doesn't usually mean a rheumatologist or an orthodox allergist. I've already explained how the arthritis establishment views nutrition and anything deriving from it, from vitamins to food allergy. That leaves the allergist and leads to a question: why won't *any* such practitioner help you to fix a possible role of allergy in arthritis? The answer is complex, but to put it oversimply, most orthodox allergists are victims of a kind of training which makes it intellectually impossible for them to accept food allergy, addictive allergy, or any other kind that doesn't involve the immune system of the body. The kinds of allergy we are discussing definitely don't involve that system, but they still make people sick, and people still get better when the offending foods are deleted from their menus. Without involvement of the immune system, food allergies still cause mental symptoms for which people are, mistakenly, treated with psychiatric conversation and calmative drugs. They still cause colds, bronchitis, asthma, fatigability, irritability, neurotic behavior, diarrhea, constipation, and persistent disturbances of every organ, tissue, bone, and function of the body. The worst part of the closed medical mind in this matter of nonimmunological allergy is the fate of the patients—subjected to drugs, surgery, or psychiatry they don't need or denied potential help for arthritis, with which, they are told, they must learn to live.

I am often asked whether an aversion to a food—certainly the antithesis of addictive allergic craving—could betoken allergy to that food. In children under two years of age, a marked aversion is a pretty fair indicator of allergy, and should be respected. In older children and in adults, it is obvious that such a voice of inner wisdom is rare, for if it were common, no one would be addicted to the foods to which he is allergic. This doesn't bar an aversion's meriting study, for it may be based on a vague—virtually subconscious—realization that indulgence in the disliked food subtly dilutes one's sense of well-being, or causes indigestion, headache, increased muscle stiffness, joint pain, or other symptoms. But the value of an adult's aversions is diminished by other possibilities. For example, the dislike of many people for foods in the cabbage family isn't predicated on allergy, but derives from a genetic tendency to taste such foods as bitter.

Mentioning the cabbage family reminds you again that there are biological families into which foods fall, where allergy to one member of a biological group brings up the strong possibility of allergy to one or more of the others. Thus an allergy to soy would increase the likelihood of allergy to other legumes, such as peas. Some of the relationships defy the layman's logic: chamomile, an herb tea long used for infant colic, is biologically related to ragweed, which could mean that the person with hay fever might touch off his arthritic aches and pains by drinking that herb tea. For this reason, I have provided you, in the Appendix, with both alphabetical and numerical listings of foods and their family relationships.

It should be emphasized that frequency or infrequency of eating an allergenic food would not be the only variable in altering its effect on an allergic person. Cooking may eliminate, lessen, or increase your reactivity to foods to which you are sensitive. There are those who can't eat onions cooked in an open pot but tolerate those cooked under a cover. There are people who can't eat onions raw but suffer no ill effects if the vegetable has been previously soaked in vinegar. Some can't eat coleslaw but tolerate cooked cabbage. The person allergic to ordinary pasteurized milk may have no difficulty with certified raw milk. Those who react to both forms of milk may have no trouble if it has been brought to a boil and promptly chilled. Some can't endure milk but have no problem with cheese. Sometimes it makes a difference if the cheese is highly fermented, like a cheddar, as against the less fermented, like cottage or pot cheese. Then there are people who tolerate acidophilus milk, kefir, or yogurt, but suffer if they drink ordinary milk. Quantity may make as much of a difference as frequency of consumption.

To this point, we've dealt only with methods, old and new, of tracking down the allergies which may be present and may be worsening your arthritis, tendonitis, muscle spasms, or other source of pain, swelling, and stiffness. Let me make sure that I've left no doubt that an allergy hunt is worthwhile for an arthritic. Apart from those whom I've seen benefited by identification of allergies and removal of the insults from the internal and external environments (food, chemicals, etc.), there is the simple, unequivocal statement I've heard from a number of avant-garde allergists who have investigated the link between food sensitivities and arthritic diseases. Among these are Dr. Marshall Mandell, Dr. Robert Stroud, and Dr. Theron Randolph, and among their comments were such statements as:

1. Sixty-seven percent of arthritics examined in one study actually had an allergy-related disease which could be relieved by removing offending foods from the diet and controlling external factors, such as household dust.
2. In overall surveys of arthritics on usual medications, an allergist reported that the drugs could be stopped for more than 50 percent of the patients when the offending foods were removed from their menus.
3. Dr. Stroud commented that he, as a rheumatologist, has concluded that "an important number of patients with rheumatoid arthritis and osteoarthritis are responding to elimination of food from their diet."

4. Dr. Randolph, dean of bioecological allergy in this country, remarked vis-a-vis the benefits of identifying and removing allergens from the patient's diet and environment: "Not only can we relieve untold suffering, but prevent a great deal of undesirable side effects from drugs."

Bioecological allergists are few in number, and orthodox allergy societies ignore them, their philosophy, and their findings, exactly as they ignored Dr. Coca's research. In the Appendix, you will find suggestions for locating such practitioners, as well as medical nutritionists, orthomolecular psychiatrists, and others who are practicing the medicine and the nutrition of tomorrow. That doesn't mean that a practitioner will be available in your community, or, for that matter, in your state. There are only a few hundred of these avant-garde allergists, and it may be necessary to travel to visit one. I can only repeat that the effort has been rewarding for some arthritics—meaning those whose allergies and arthritis turned out to be related. Before you act on a referral, it is important to query the physician to be sure that his investigations of bioecological allergy are directed toward the problem in which you are interested. There are bioecological allergists who are pediatricians, others who are psychiatrists, and some who are devoted to research rather than clinical practice; none of these, obviously, would be the physician of choice for an adult arthritic.

Diagnosing allergy, despite the concentrated efforts it demands, would seem to be easier than lessening or eliminating it, as you might conclude from the discussion to this point, for it has apparently given you only three resources to help you to cope with allergy once you've identified it:

1. The desensitization injections, such as are given to hay fever sufferers.
2. Abstaining totally from contact, internal or external, with foods, drugs, or chemicals to which you are allergic.

3. Lengthening the intervals between exposures to foods to which you are sensitive—exemplified in the rotation diet. It is based on the observation that infrequency of exposure to offending foods gives the body rest periods in which to build its defences.

There remain to be discussed other ways of reducing the severity of allergies. These include neutralizing doses, vitamin and diet therapy, and correction of metabolic disturbances, like hypoglycemia, which may initiate or worsen allergic reactions. All these approaches have a common denominator: they are frequently helpful to some patients, even those with aggravated allergic tendencies, and they are rarely used in the orthodox management of allergies.

In describing neutralizing doses, I want to emphasize that no one really understands why this simple technique is often very effective in controlling addictive craving for allergenic foods and in reducing or canceling allergic reactions. But lack of understanding why it works is no excuse for bypassing its possible benefits. We don't understand all the actions of aspirin, but that hasn't stopped us from swallowing tons of it, has it?

3

Nutritional Helps for Allergic Arthritics

NEUTRALIZING DOSES

Let's assume one of your principal troublemakers is milk. Your craving for it is strong, your withdrawal symptoms are unbearable, and drinking a glassful gives you enough temporary relief (the "high") to keep you addicted. We are going to search for a neutralizing dose, which might be one, two, three, or more drops of milk in a quarter of a glass of water. We'll know which is the proper dose when it cancels your craving and most, if not all, of your withdrawal symptoms. Solid foods like meat can be tested by swallowing a minute amount, perhaps the size of the head of a pin, and gradually increasing the test dose. Foods which are soluble—like sugar—can of course be appropriately diluted in water for testing. Cereals, breads, and the like can be soaked in water for hours and a drop of that solution in water used as the starting test dose. There are opportunities, of course, for this type of testing to fail. You may not identify the correct neutralizing dose. You may not respond—some people don't —to any dose. You may fail because there is a contaminant in the food to which you are sensitive, and for which the neutralizing dose of the food itself isn't correct. Example: the milk you are testing may contain traces of pesticides; many foods do. Finally, the test may be thrown off because the water itself contains contaminants. This makes it advisable to eliminate that variable by testing with a water you know to be pure—distilled water, for example.

Bioecological allergists usually search for a neutralizing dose by giving a shallow injection of the food. Their literature, to my knowledge, does not indicate that they have explored the possibility of establishing such doses by oral administration of the food. I believe, after watching doses by mouth give striking relief in some cases, that this method deserves more investigation.

In establishing neutralizing doses by injection, the bioecological allergist and the medical nutritionist often employ vaccines by a method which converts the vaccine from a preventive measure to one which is a treatment. Influenza vaccine is a good example. Ordinarily, one takes an injection of this drug only in the effort to prevent or at least to minimize influenza if it strikes. The allergists greatly dilute the vaccine, and give varying but minute doses. When they strike the right one, it is effective even for a patient who already has influenza, for it will wipe out the symptoms, or greatly reduce them, in as little as a half hour; moreover, that dose can be given again, with the same good results, if the patient has another attack of the virus. These results parallel those obtained with neutralizing doses of foods and other allergens, though I must again call to your attention that the reports in the literature deal with injections rather than oral doses. I am not apologizing for making what appears to be a unique observation, but I don't want your physician vainly searching research reports on desensitization by oral dosage.

Actually, there is no logical reason why neutralizing doses by mouth can't be established. After all, the physician uses the mouth—under the tongue, as I've explained, as a means of testing allergic reactions—and the same route logically should be effective in establishing a neutralizing dose. And that brings us to the resources of the nutritionist in helping the arthritic—not only with his allergies but, as you will learn later, in direct treatment of this group of painful diseases.

VITAMIN AND DIET THERAPY

Rheumatologists ignore nutrition for reasons you now understand, but why do allergists? And they do ignore it: only recently they have been scolded for making no effort to teach patients to compensate for dietary inadequacies caused by a long list of forbidden foods. As for treatment of allergies with nutritional therapies, it is as if it doesn't exist, though anyone conversant with the scientific literature can quote a number of reports on benefits to the allergic from special dietary procedures or vitamin therapies.

A typical example is an experiment in the treatment of twenty-five patients with so many allergies that their diets were critically restricted. The physician began, in the traditional way of medical research, with experiments on animals, and what he learned promised—and delivered—benefits to his human patients. He first gave the animals injections of a sensitizing substance to initiate a tendency to allergy toward it. He followed that, weeks later, with second injections of the substance, which in most of the animals created an allergic reaction so violent that it was lethal. He repeated that experiment with a second group of animals, but intervened between the first and second injections with various medications, among which were nutrients. Ultimately, he found that supplements of Vitamin B Complex and protein were strikingly effective in reducing the severity of the allergic reaction to the second series of injections. He then transferred the principle to his twenty-five highly allergic patients, giving them predigested protein* and what he called

*Predigested protein usually no longer has the alergenic properties specific to its source. Thus predigested milk protein is unlikely to cause allergic reactions in patients sensitive to milk, and this applies to protein from other sources, so treated. Products of this kind were commercially available for many years, but appear to be disappearing from the market. The physician can, of course, substitute concentrates of any high-quality protein to which the patient is not sensitive. Rotation of sources would then be prudent.

a "Vitamin B Complex cocktail." In two years of that treatment, twenty-two of the twenty-five patients responded as the animals had, with a lessening of allergy to the point where restrictions on their diets could be lifted. And when, in introducing this discussion, I remarked that allergists ignore nutritional therapies as if they didn't exist, I meant it: in some thirty-five years as a nutrition educator for both the public and the professions, I have never met an allergist who read the report I just reviewed for you. (It appeared in the *Annals of Allergy*, an A.M.A. publication.)

Another report that went largely unnoticed derived from an experiment in the administration of Vitamin B_{12} to malnourished children who were not growing normally. Striking growth responses were encountered, of which the most startling was that of a little boy who grew nearly six inches in two years of administration of the vitamin. Although the report came from a distinguished pediatrician, and appeared in an establishment journal, it was ignored. So was the fact that the little boy's asthma disappeared in the course of the vitamin treatment. It may well be that the improvement in the child's asthma will rarely (or never) be matched in other victims of an allergic asthma, but we'll never know, because this report, too, has been gathering dust in the medical libraries. And we aren't likely to discover what the vitamin will or won't do for arthritics whose aches and pains are being fanned by allergy.

What I have just written could have been directed to Vitamin E therapy, or treatment with Vitamin C, for both factors have been used successfully in the treatment of hay fever. (Vitamins E and C have other helpful actions in arthritis, directly, which will be discussed later.) Action in hay fever raises the possibility of helpfulness in other types of allergies which may be part of the problems of the arthritic.

Vitamin B_{12} is usually given by injection, because absorption of the vitamin when taken by mouth is poor even in patients with efficient digestive tracts. In those lacking sufficient stomach hydrochloric acid, or deficient in internal production of a cofactor (intrinsic factor) needed for absorption, utilization of the vitamin when given by mouth may be at best unpredictable. A recent development offers a useful compromise, in the form of lozenges of the vitamin for sublingual (under-the-tongue) absorption. When these are dissolved under the tongue, the vitamin is absorbed directly by the rich circulation of blood there, which thereby detours the digestive tract. The principle is the same as that physicians utilize when they instruct heart patients to dissolve nitroglycerin tablets under the tongue. The B_{12} lozenges are available in potencies as high as 500 micrograms, and physicians seeking saturation with the vitamin may prescribe six, eight, or more daily. The treatment with Vitamin B_{12} may be a component of a more comprehensive therapy for such disorders as bursitis, with ultrasonic therapy also used.

Large doses of Vitamin C are used in the management of allergies, as well as in such arthritic disorders as rheumatoid arthritis and ankylosing spondylitis. The scare stories about drastic side effects of Vitamin C are scares and nothing more, predicated upon theoretical chemistries which these critics, usually professional "antinutrition" propagandists, who never attack the dangerous drugs freely prescribed, can't verify in human beings. There is one common side reaction to Vitamin C when used in large doses: diarrhea. Far from being a deterrent to the use of the vitamin, the reaction is utilized by medical nutritionists to establish the highest dose the patients can tolerate: i.e., if diarrhea eventuates, the dose which causes it establishes the dose beneath it, which will not cause diarrhea. Another way of circumventing the problem is the use of sustained-release forms of Vitamin C, which permit maintenance of elevated blood levels of the vitamin without the need for massive oral doses. The usual form of sustained-release tablets comprises little pellets of the vitamin, which are resin coated, forcing the body to strip the coating before the vitamin can be released. The variabilities of human digestive functions being what they are, the release of the vitamin may be capricious, or at least unpredictable, with this type of formulation. Another, which I consider superior, has the pellets of the vitamin mechanically seated in a matrix, from which the body must extract the vitamin. I have seen blood-level determinations which indicated that this will yield more consistent blood levels of Vitamin C than the resin-coated formulations. The sustained-release preparations, of whatever type, are often prescribed in but two doses daily—perhaps on arising and before retiring—unless the physician is seeking markedly high blood levels of the vitamin.

Vitamin B_6, which as you will learn later is markedly helpful in a type of arthritis, also has an antiallergy effect when administered with Vitamin C. The two nutrients have proved very useful to bioecological allergists and medical nutritionists, as well as orthomolecular psychiatrists, in the treatment of cerebral allergies. These are allergic reactions which affect the brain, though they may not cause any of the symptoms of conventional allergy, and thereby induce behavior which may range from depression to outright psychosis. Since allergy as a factor in arthritis has received little attention, this vitamin combination has not been tested, as it should be, for what it can do for the allergic arthritic. I can tell you, from actual observation, that the combination has not only been useful as a treatment for such allergic symptoms, but as prevention; and I am not writing about cerebral allergy alone. As an example, in individuals with marked allergic reactivity to dust and pollen, large doses of Vitamin C and Vitamin B_6, taken both before and after exposure to these allergens, have markedly mitigated or sometimes totally blocked the allergic reaction. Both of these nutrients affect the immune system, which is known to be disturbed in rheumatoid arthritis, and one might anticipate usefulness for these vitamins for people with that form of arthritis, as well as for those whose allergies are a component of their problems with other types of the disease. Physicians may recommend one gram (1,000 milligrams) of each vitamin, always taken together, as treatment for allergic symptoms, and lesser amounts to be used when exposure to an allergen is anticipated and unavoidable. A typical example of the unavoidable would be eating in a restaurant, where recipes are filled with question marks. Allergic to corn, you avoid corn on the cob, but may fall prey to the cornstarch concealed in the gravy. For those whose allergic symptoms respond to Vitamins B_6 and C, these nutrients become a first-aid kit protecting against the unavoidable.

The bioflavonoids are a group of nutritional factors which have three actions useful to the allergic arthritic. The group includes citrus bioflavonoids, rutin, hesperidin, and herperidin chalcone. Which of these may be useful will be in part determined by the presence or absence of allergy to citrus fruits, which may bar the use of the bioflavonoids from such sources, in which case the other types can be used. The most effective types appear to be the citrus bioflavonoids and the hesperidin types. Rutin is less soluble, and may thereby be less effective. All these factors reduce excessive permeability of the walls of the small blood vessels, and all strengthen the vessels. Excessive permeability is responsible for the loss of fluid which creates the watery eyes and the boggy, soggy, water-laden tissues of the nose which mark pollen allergy. More directly of interest to the allergic arthritic is the fact that the bioflavonoids may by this action help to reduce abnormal collections of fluid in the joints. They have, for instance, helped bursitis.

These factors also help to protect Vitamin C against oxidation in the body, thereby making the vitamin more effective. There is evidence, too, that they may reduce the intensity of the allergic process, exactly as did the Vitamin B Complex and protein supplements discussed earlier. It has long bothered me that supplementary and therapeutic doses of the bioflavonoids have been low, too low, sometimes, for effectiveness. If one realizes that an orange may supply nine times as much of the bioflavonoids as of Vitamin C, it doesn't make sense that Vitamin C doses have been greatly escalated—in some therapeutic uses, as high as 160,000 milligrams daily—while the bioflavonoid intake has been held to a few hundred milligrams. Given tolerance for the factors, I see no point in supplements of less than 3 grams (3,000 milligrams) of bioflavonoids daily.

Vitamin E is virtually a specific medication for a painful muscle disorder, intermittent claudication, which for some arthritics adds to their burden of troubles. Like PABA, one of the B Complex factors, Vitamin E has a sparing effect on cortisone, allowing the physician to minimize side effects by reducing doses of this potent drug, if he must use it. It will be of interest for you to know that such a use of Vitamin E or PABA is only one example of helpful interactions between nutrients and drugs that are often not capitalized upon. For example, aspirin doses may be reduced by combining copper with the drug or by giving PABA with it. Similarly, penicillamine, a potent medication used for rheumatoid arthritis which has so many major side reactions that a large percentage of patients simply can't tolerate it, may be tamed significantly if trace minerals, magnesium, and antioxidants, such as Vitamin C and Vitamin E, are administered simultaneously. However, until the medical establishment is more receptive to (and better educated in) nutritional chemistries, these helpful combinations of nutrients and drugs aren't likely to be prescribed.

Pantothenic acid, another B Complex vitamin, sometimes described on labels as pantothenol or as calcium pantothenate (all forms of the same vitamin), has shown significant antistress, antiallergy, and antiarthritis actions. Some arthritics can't tolerate more than thirty milligrams daily, but gauging the response by the blood levels of eosinophils, which tend to rise when the body is under stress (such as allergy) and fall with large doses of pantothenic acid, physicians are using as much as one gram (1,000 milligrams) daily for patients who tolerate that amount. Such responses, both in stress and in allergy, indicate that the vitamin stimulates adrenal function. The adrenals secrete powerful antiallergy hormones, such as cortisone and adrenalin (epinephrin). The actions of the vitamin indicate that it may be directly helpful in rheumatoid arthritis, as well as in any type of arthritis where allergy is a factor. Uneven production of adrenal hormones, one theory has it, may be responsible for rheumatoid arthritis. Pantothenic acid has also been found directly helpful to allergic individuals, in reports by the scientist who first isolated and synthesized the vitamin. He is Dr. Roger Williams, who repeatedly has urged more study of the helpful actions of pantothenic acid in disease, and more investigation of the benefits of an intake far above the level most diets yield. I have heard Dr. Williams repeatedly criticize our intake of the vitamin as insufficient to support best health, and certainly inadequate to meet the needs of people with health problems. Since there are studies indicating the importance of the vitamin to adrenal function, which is critical to people with allergies and arthritis, it gives one pause to realize that pantothenic acid deficiency in animals will cause actual hemorrhages in the adrenal gland often accompanied, fascinatingly, by premature greying of the hair. In chapter 5, you will find a description of an interesting experiment with pantothenic acid in the treatment of rheumatoid arthritis. The treatment was beneficial, but try to find an orthodox rheumatologist who has (a) read the paper, which appeared in *Lancet*, a conservative medical journal, or (b) ever tried the daring experiment of giving a rheumatoid arthritic doses of the vitamin as a substitute for or an adjunct to the standard (and dangerous) hormone and drug therapies.

None of the preceding statements should be allowed to obscure the fact that supplements of vitamins, minerals, or other concentrated nutrients *are* supplements, not *sub-stitutes* for the best possible diet. I emphasize that because I am something of an authority on the tendency of the public to use supplements as licenses for eating improperly, the conventional excuse being: "It doesn't matter if I eat junk—I take my vitamins." My Ph.D. dissertation explored that point, and found that a majority of *nutrition-minded* adults who achieved adequate intake of vitamins and minerals did so despite poor diets, thanks to their use of supplements. In the classrooms of the universities and colleges, some six of them, where I have for years taught basic and advanced nutrition, assays of students' diets, assigned to them in lieu of midsemester examinations, have repeatedly demonstrated that supplements are being used to achieve nutritional adequacy not provided by their menus. Since there are many factors in foods which are not yet firmly identified, no supplement can be regarded as a substitute for a good diet. I write that in terms of healthy individuals, and emphasize it even more strongly for those who are ill, for their nutritional needs for recovery are greater than those for maintenance of good health. All this has a pointed meaning for the arthritic and even more so for the allergic arthritic, who vitally need diets aimed at meeting their individual needs. This is basic to any nutritional therapy, and the therapy itself must be undertaken as early as possible and must be complete, concentrated, consistent, and continuous.

All this by way of preface to our next subject: diets for arthritis. Note the plural—not *the* diet for arthritis. It isn't one disease; there isn't one diet. And even in considering the feeding of two patients with the same type of arthritis, there still isn't one diet which can be recommended. For nutritional requirements and tolerances aren't standardized, any more than people are. And the impact of a disease on a patient is only half the story; there is also the impact of the patient on the disease.

4

Your Meals and
Your Arthritis

When millions of people suffer with one variety of arthritis or another, and treatment is largely symptomatic and thereby unsatisfactory, it's inevitable that various types of diets or foods will be blamed for the diseases, and others credited with controlling or curing them. Much of this is nothing more than folklore, and offers the Arthritis Foundation an opportunity periodically to inveigh against nutrition quackery. Such campaigns are really an indictment of the failure of the orthodoxy to find causes or cures for this group of diseases, and tend to obscure the genuinely valuable nutritional therapies.

So it is that vegetarians insist that too much protein—which their diets almost never could supply—is *the* cause of arthritis, making vegetarianism sovereign prevention and a sure cure, though that should mean that all herbivorous animals should escape the disease (they don't), all carnivorous animals should suffer with it (they don't), and human vegetarians should never develop it (they sometimes do).

Enthusiasts for natural foods place the blame on everything from pesticide residues in food to food additives and overprocessing, though man endured arthritis long before General Mills and Kellogg raped the grain and salted it with questionable preservatives. Not only do the bones of dinosaurs show the marks of arthritis, but they are also apparent in X-ray examinations of some Egyptian mummies, and history records that the American Indian complained of pain in his joints, and the Crusaders were sometimes immobilized by arthritis. Neanderthal man didn't escape. Neither did the little eohippus, the ultimate ancestor of the horse. And while arthritics journey to Tucson to seek the benefits of its climate, there are Arizonans who come to New York for treatment.

All this I tell you to put in proper perspective those who point to a single specific factor in our diets or our way of life as *the* cause of arthritis. Aware of the risk of that kind of thinking is the famous publisher who has told the inspiring story of his recovery from ankylosing spondylitis, ordinarily a progressively crippling disorder, by the use of massive doses of Vitamin C, laughter, and exercise. He doesn't propose that regime as a panacea, knowing full well that the next patient might respond less or perhaps not at all. Actually, I'd expect laughter—or more precisely, the patient's emotional state—to play a greater role in rheumatoid arthritis, where the immune system, which is exquisitely sensitive to the emotions, is known to be deranged. (There is, in fact, at least one study of rheumatoid arthritics which indicates that a striking percentage of these patients are unhappy with themselves, their life roles, and their accomplishments.)

As for massive doses of Vitamin C, helpful in many disorders, from hepatitis to drug addiction, I'm reminded that some of the no-nightshade dieters who were benefited by avoiding those foods reported adverse effects from large doses of the vitamin. Dr. Childers attributes this to an intolerance to the vitamin itself, but since these individuals may tolerate the vitamin from natural sources, such as citrus fruit, it is possible that the adverse reaction represents an allergy to the source of the synthetic vitamin, which is corn, a food to which many people are allergic. Don't let that statement startle you: there are people who react to cane sugar, but not to beet sugar. Sugar is sugar, but the source counts, just as alcohol is alcohol, but some people react to rye who are not bothered by Scotch, the source being the obvious variable.

Dr. Dong, a Chinese physician practicing in the United States, developed a severe and crippling arthritis, and ultimately traced it to his reaction to the typical American diet. He recovered when he returned to ancestral Chinese menus, emphasizing seafood and vegetables, and applied these findings to many arthritic patients, with fine results. Yet I have seen arthritics who recovered when placed on a well-balanced diet comprising typical American selections of foods, with fairly high intake of animal proteins, sans emphasis on seafoods, and only nominal intake of fruits and vegetables. By the same token, the low-fat, high-carbohydrate, low-protein meals of the Central African type, theorized by Nathan Pritikin as virtual panaceas for prevention and treatment of diseases of civilization, could be a fertile source of potential troubles for rheumatoid arthritics. (As I write that, I am thinking of Dr. Weston A. Price, who records, in *Nutrition and Physical Degeneration* (La Mesa, Calif.: Price-Pottenger, 1977), the history of a little boy with Still's disease—juvenile rheumatoid arthritis—who was converted from a helpless little cripple into a healthier and happier youngster by Price's diet, which placed special emphasis on a high intake of good-quality butter. I am also thinking of another child, with rheumatic fever, whose physician called me for a nutritional consultation. I recommended four eggs—the opposite of the Pritikin diet—daily. Seven years later, that youngster was well enough to serve in the armed forces.)

What I have just written reflects a philosophy of nutrition which recognizes that we are all individuals, that our differences are greater than our similarities, and that nutritional needs and tolerances differ as much as people themselves do. That is really what we're citing when we indict allergy as a neglected factor in arthritis, for allergy is simply individual differences gone berserk, so that one man's meat (or fish or fowl or vegetable) is another man's poison. This is not the same process involved in intolerance to the nightshades, which rests more upon toxic than on allergic effects. It is also not necessarily the same process involved in sensitivity to sugar, which can be responsible for simulating or aggravating arthritis via hypoglycemia (low blood sugar), a disorder which appears to combine the worst features of toxicity and allergy, superimposed upon malnutrition. As a factor in some considerable number of cases of arthritis, hypoglycemia is neglected as is allergy, which is ironic, for it can cause or aggravate allergy, too, making the threat a double one. It was important that you understand the contributions of nightshade intolerance and food allergies to arthritis. It is just as important that you become familiar with another (neglected) problem for arthritics: low blood sugar (hypoglycemia).

Medical reactionaries, like those of the AMA, have trumpeted their belief that low blood sugar is a fad disease, utilized by hypochondriacs to escape the psychiatric treatment they need and exploited by physicians who are venal, incompetent, or both. The AMA's penchant for talking out of both sides of its mouth was never better illustrated than in this antihypoglycemia campaign, for while these warnings were reaching the public, the medical society was busy giving a course for physicians in diagnosis and treatment of the "fad" disease. In the event that you have encountered that kind of propaganda, let me briefly note that the Institute for Child Development diagnosed hypoglycemia in 60 percent of two hundred hyperactive children treated by them; Farris found it in 14 percent of five thousand young GI's previously labeled healthy; and United Airlines discovered that 44 of 177 pilots (forty years of age and older) suffered with it. Unamusingly, when I lectured on the subject to United Airlines personnel, and asked one of the pilots what his hypoglycemic symptoms were, he replied: "Nothing much— just in driving a car in heavy traffic, I would feel confused, and have to pull over to the side and rest for a while!"

I myself have acted as an educator and a consultant to hundreds of physicians who daily encounter hypoglycemia, previously unrecognized and, of course, thereby untreated, among patients in their practices. But these are medical nutritionists for the most part, who have a high index of suspicion for the condition and are aware of the ways in which it will mimic or intensify physical disease and how it is capable of making an emotional and mental wreck out of an otherwise normal person. They also know how to test for low blood sugar and how properly to interpret the results of the tests. In that sentence is buried another frustration for the nutrition educator, for the orthodox standards for "normal" and "low" blood sugars are often completely arbitrary and completely misleading. For one thing, how normal are "norms" derived from a population which eats more than one hundred pounds of sugar per capita, per year, a dietary insult which evokes abnormal reactions in 20 percent of the population, according to the Carbohydrate Laboratory of the U.S. Department of Agriculture?

To comprehend what low blood sugar can do, not only in worsening arthritis and its symptoms but in wrecking you physically and mentally, I present here the lists of symptoms reported by 1,100 patients treated by Stephen Gyland, M.D., and those of an additional 1,300 patients treated by my research colleague, Dr. Herman Goodman. This is so arranged that it becomes a home test for possible hypoglycemia. You will note that the symptoms are presented in two lists. You can score your results yourself by writing yes or no after each item and then multiplying each "yes" answer in column 1 by 3 and each "yes" answer in column 2 by 2. Add the two totals. If the score is over 58, our experience indicates that you should see a medical nutritionist, for there will be a strong possibility that you have hypoglycemia, which will mean that there is an equally strong possibility that it is making worse your aches, stiffness, pains, and lack of energy.

COLUMN 1

Nervousness _____
Irritability _____
Depression _____
Forgetfulness _____
Insomnia (Awakening in
  the small hours, unable
  to return to sleep) _____
Constant worrying _____
Mental confusion _____
Unsocial, antisocial
  behavior _____
Unprovoked crying
  spells _____
Indecisiveness _____
Lack of sexual drive
  (females) _____
Impotence (males) _____
Night terrors,
  nightmares _____
Phobias, fears _____
Suicidal thoughts _____
Restlessness _____
Nervous breakdowns _____

  Total "yes" answers _____
  Multiplied by 3 _____

COLUMN 2

Exhaustion _____
Faintness, tremors, cold
  sweats, weak spells _____
Vertigo (dizziness or
  sensations of falling) _____
Drowsiness _____
Headaches _____
Chronic indigestion _____
A feeling of internal
  trembling _____
Palpitation of the heart _____
Rapid pulse _____
Muscle pain _____
Numbness _____
Allergies _____
Incoordination _____
Leg cramps _____
Blurred vision _____
Twitching, jerking,
  cramping of leg
  muscles _____
Itching and crawling
  sensations on skin _____
Gasping for breath _____
Smothering spells _____
Staggering _____
Episodes of blackout or
  unconsciousness _____
Rheumatoid arthritis _____
Neurodermatitis _____
Lack of appetite _____
Compulsive craving for
  sweets, colas, coffee, tea,
  chocolate _____
Joint pains _____
Abdominal spasms _____
Obesity _____
Underweight _____
Compulsive drinking of
  alcoholic beverages _____

  Total "yes" answers _____
  Multiplied by 2 _____

Combined totals, columns 1 and 2 _____

As you answered the questions, it must have occurred to you that a number of symptoms which hypoglycemics suffer are identical with those which arthritics often exhibit—including numbness, leg cramps, joint pains, and twitching and jerking of leg muscles. There is nothing, of course, to prevent such symptoms from being caused by arthritis itself, but they can also be initiated or aggravated by hypoglycemia. It may be of interest for you to know what percentages of these thousands of hypoglycemics complained of symptoms common in arthritics. Fifty-three percent of them cited muscle pains. Fifty-one percent listed numbness as a problem. Leg cramps appeared in 43 percent of the patients with low blood sugar. Forty-three percent, incidentally, underscored the relationship between hypoglycemia and allergies by noting allergic symptoms as a problem. Twitching and jerking of the muscles afflicted 39 percent. And rheumatoid arthritis (which wasn't rheumatoid arthritis, but a penalty for low blood sugar) was the complaint of 24 percent. All these symptoms, including the "rheumatoid arthritis," were diminished sharply or disappeared when the hypoglycemia was brought under control. Many of these patients had been told that they were hypochondriacs or neurotics, diagnoses as far off target as was the verdict of rheumatoid arthritis for one in fourteen of these hypoglycemics.

Let me emphasize that I don't want to kindle the hope that your arthritis is nothing more than the product of an unrecognized low blood sugar or, for that matter, an unrecognized penalty for allergies. On the other hand, the chances range from one in ten to one in twenty—depending on the educated guesses at the incidence of low blood sugar—that it may be worsening your arthritis and initiating other disorders and other symptoms. It has been said that virus infections have great efficiency in making preexisting health problems worse. This is true, but viruses share that capability with hypoglycemia and allergies, which can trap you in a very vicious circle, for low blood sugar can start the allergic process or worsen it, and is the end point of a diet and lifestyle which can make you more subject to viral and other infections. While a study of the symptoms reported by thousands of hypoglycemics is certainly a firm basis for drawing conclusions, there is even stronger evidence for the statistical probability that your aches and pains are being fanned by low blood sugar. That evidence surfaced in 1980, when the Carbohydrate Laboratory of the Agriculture Department studied the reactions of average Americans to our average intake of sugar, from which we draw 18 percent of our calories. That level causes adverse physiological reactions which were characteristic of 20 percent of American men. (This doesn't exclude women—only male volunteers participated in the study.) And we have long known that disturbances of carbohydrate (starch-sugar) metabolism are found in rheumatoid arthritics as well as in a number of other serious disorders, including cancer.

All this is intended to justify asking you to read carefully what follows, which is an explanation of hypoglycemia— how it begins, and precisely what it does to you. Although low blood sugar sounds like a minor problem with a simplistic solution—eating more sugar—it is a complicated disorder, made worse by eating more sugar, for it represents an inability of the body to cope with the excessive intake of that empty food. Moreover, the roots of hypoglycemia are found in the combined effects of stress, caffeine, allergies, and malnutrition.

Every twenty seconds, approximately, the brain completes a very long series of chemical reactions (the Krebs cycle) by which glucose (sugar) is transformed into energy. So dependent is the brain on an adequate supply of glucose that there is no threshold for its entrance to the brain from the blood. In other words, there is no point at which the body will block admission of blood sugar to the brain, though it is highly selective of both the substances and the amounts of them which are permitted to pass the barrier between the blood and the brain. The vital dependence of the brain on a continuous, adequate supply of this preferred fuel is apparent when one considers the irritability, nervousness, fatigue, or headaches which some people suffer when deprived of a meal or two. The individual difference which creates penalties for meal-skipping in *some* people, but not all, is the kind of difference which creates low blood sugar in some people and, under the same circumstances, not in others. To put it in the language of one of the physicians who attended my medical seminars on hypoglycemia: "I learned that a hypoglycemic is a person who can't stand small fluctuations in blood sugar levels which don't bother the rest of us." He was responding to an effort by the profession to set a "magic number"—a level of blood sugar which marks the borderline between normalcy and low blood sugar. There is no such invariant number. There are only people with very variable reactions to changes in the internal environment, and among these, a group very sensitive to the effects of stress garnished with a poor diet high in sugar and in caffeine. These become the hypoglycemics. They also become the derelicts of orthodox medicine, for three reasons:

1. They have so many symptoms that they must appear to be hypochondriacs or neurotics.
2. The medical test for low blood sugar, unlike that for diabetes, requires six hours and is therefore not likely to be routine in a "complete physical examination."
3. If the test is given by a physician indoctrinated by the orthodoxy, he will look for the "magic number" and, failing to find it, will assure the patient that he's normal.

Consider number 3 carefully. Should the patient actually be hypoglycemic, despite passing the "magic number" criterion, and should all the other test results be reasonably normal, what do you think the physician will conclude about this "well patient" who is complaining about weakness, unprovoked crying, inexplicable depression and suicidal thoughts, great fatigue, craving for sweets, muscle pains, impotence or frigidity, insomnia, and indigestion so severe that it suggests a stomach ulcer—which isn't there? You've guessed it: he'll call it hypochondriasis, neurosis, psychoneurosis, or in very aggravated cases, psychosis. And the patient will be offered tranquilizers, psychiatric treatment, or both. And make no mistake about what I'm telling you: that is the documented history of thousands of hypoglycemics, because of the traditional resistance of medicine both to nutrition and to new ideas. Should you be an arthritic with low blood sugar, do you think you'll fare any better? Not unless you escape the orthodox rheumatologist or internist, and find a physician—who will probably be a medical nutritionist—with a high index of suspicion for low blood sugar.

What happens when blood sugar drops is dramatically emphasized when a diabetic takes an overdose of insulin, the hormone needed to burn sugar, and falls unconscious. Question: is it possible for a person who isn't diabetic, and isn't taking insulin, to produce an overdose of insulin, manufactured within the body? Why not? The pancreas, where insulin is manufactured, is a gland, and any gland in the body can become overactive. Dozens of disorders are traced to glands gone wild; why should the pancreas be an exception? The fact that it isn't was recognized more than fifty years ago, when hypoglycemia was first reported. Ironically, the physician who discovered hypoglycemia resulting from excessive production of insulin was given a gold medal by the AMA—which now calls it an imaginary disease.

We have now identified one of many causes of hypoglycemia; it happens to be the most common one: an excessive insulin response to a sudden rise in blood sugar. (In a diabetic, it's called "insulin shock.") Two factors in the

diet can cause the blood sugar to rise too quickly: sugar
itself, and caffeine, which stimulates the adrenal glands into
producing hormones which raise the blood sugar. (That's
why reducers get a lift from black coffee. Its caffeine causes
a release of stored blood sugar, which enters the blood.) To
the blood sugar rise, the body responds by producing insulin
to burn off the excess glucose. If the insulin response is excessive, a vicious cycle develops: eating sugar actually *lowers* blood sugar (after a brief initial rise). The "wisdom of the
body," unable to cope with the abnormal situation, may respond by creating a "sweet tooth." Satisfying that craving
starts the whole process all over again. This, in fact, can also
explain the obese person who greedily swallows candy, complaining that the more he eats, the more he wants. It is also
an explanation of a type of asthma, a type of alcoholism, and
other disorders in which hypoglycemia is sometimes im-
plicated, but those are beyond the scope of this book.*

There is no function, no organ in the body which isn't
adversely affected by lack of fuel. Disturbances of the brain
and nervous systems result from hypoglycemia, with dramatic effects at three different levels. The emotional brain is
exquisitely sensitive to low blood sugar, and reacts as if a
panic button had been pushed—which actually it has—creating restlessness or zestlessness, irritability, depression unrelated to the life situation, anxiety, phobias, weeping without apparent cause, claustrophobia, and other "emotional"
symptoms. The thinking brain doesn't escape, with symptoms ranging from shortening of the memory and attention
spans to feelings of depersonalization. The autonomic center
in the brain is an early target for the low blood sugar process. Here are the controls for the functions of the body
which ordinarily don't demand our voluntary supervision:

*Readers wishing to explore hypoglycemia in greater depth are referred to *Low
Blood Sugar and You* (New York: Grosset & Dunlap, 1969, available in hardcover
and paperback). It is the text I wrote with Dr. Herman Goodman, after many decades of research in low blood sugar.

breathing, heart rate, and digestive functions among others. So it is that hypoglycemics complain of gastric pain, of rapid pulse, of a sensation of skipped beats of the heart. Compounding the difficulties as sugar levels fall is a disturbance of blood calcium-phosphorus function, which contributes to spasm of the muscles. Those who criticize hypoglycemics as suffering from too many symptoms are surely uneducated in the anatomy, chemistry, and function of the body.

If on the basis of your self-test for hypoglycemia, or because you want to be sure that your arthritis isn't being worsened by it, you decide to go for a medical test for low blood sugar, you should understand the testing methods used. The most common is the six-hour glucose (sugar) tolerance test. You will be asked to come to the doctor's office or the laboratory without breakfast. There you will have the first (fasting) blood sugar determination. This will be followed by a large dose of sugar, usually in a flavored drink. Subsequently, depending on the individual physician's techniques, your blood sugar levels will be tested at the half-hour or one-hour interval and every hour after that, for a total of six. Two warnings: shorter tests—two, three, or four hours—may miss the condition. The disturbance may not show up that early. Second: never undergo the test without the physician, his nurse, or his assistant uninterruptedly in the room with you. Some patients discover their low blood sugar only by going into actual convulsions on the laboratory table during the course of the test. It's rare, but it has happened. A third warning: the symptoms you develop during the test, if any, are more meaningful than the numbers. That's what's wrong with the "magic number" concept, in which the physician regards hypoglycemia as being demonstrated only if the patient's blood sugar drops below 50, 40, or some other arbitrarily chosen level. If the test increases your arthritic pains, brings on muscle spasms or numbness, gives you a headache, or makes you dizzy or irritable, you should report the symptoms to your physician and he, in turn, should use your observation as a critical factor in deciding whether or not you have hypoglycemia.

Some professionals—and I am among them—dislike the glucose tolerance test just described. We may recommend it because it is time-honored and it's easier to persuade physicians to perform it than other tests. But it really doesn't examine you under normal circumstances. Normally, you don't swallow a dollop of sugar while lying supine in the peace of a laboratory. You usually take it in meals and snacks in the course of a day's activities, and there is a method of testing you under those circumstances. In it, you report for a determination of your fasting blood sugar level, before breakfast. You then eat breakfast and return for a test afterward, another in midmorning, another before and after lunch, and in midafternoon. Disadvantage: there is no way for the physician to observe any symptoms you may experience. Advantage: this test may show disturbances in sugar metabolism which will not appear if you're resting in a laboratory, free of stress. Sometimes the afternoon reading will differ sharply from those in the morning, and symptoms will similarly change.

It must have occurred to you that the acid test for low blood sugar would be a trial of the diet. The premise is uncomplicated: if you feel better on a hypoglycemia diet, you must have the disorder. This isn't a revolutionary thought, for medical men have applied it before—in gout, for instance. If the physician isn't sure that the disorder is actually gout, he'll give the patient a drug that helps gout and nothing else. If it's an effective treatment, he has made a therapeutic diagnosis. Unfortunately, however gratifying it is when the diet for low blood sugar gets rid of some of your muscle and joint pain or other symptoms, there are four possibilities to explain the response:

> 1. You had low blood sugar, and the diet controlled it.

2. You formerly were eating foods to which you were allergic, and which weren't permitted on the new diet.
3. Your problems didn't orginate with low blood sugar or with allergies, but with malnourishment, and an excellent diet obviously pulled you out of deficiencies.
4. Your problems sprang from a combination of all three possibilities—which isn't a rare occurrence—and the diet controlled low blood sugar, eliminated allergenic foods, and corrected malnutrition.

Usually, the patient doesn't give the proverbial tinker's damn about medical antipathy to treatment without preliminary confirmation of the diagnosis. The problem is, of course, finding a physician who agrees with you.

Overproduction of insulin is the working description of the cause of one type of hypoglycemia.* There are other types, including low blood sugar caused by smoking, allergy, intolerance of amino (protein) acids, cancer, and deficiency in a hormone which is an antagonist of insulin. The list is partial. The point is that my discussion is aimed at the type which is believed to be most common: hypoglycemia caused by hyper- (overproduction of) insulin. There are also variations in the type of blood sugar curve which is revealed in the glucose tolerance tests. That to which this discussion is primarily devoted is the so-called "classical" hypoglycemic curve, in which, following an oral dose of sugar, the curve mounts steeply, then drops too rapidly. There is another type of response, called a flat curve, in

*Elevated blood insulin levels, incidentally, may not cause low blood sugar, but can cause exactly the same symptoms, which may include emotional and mental disturbances, or digestive pain suggesting the presence of a stomach ulcer—which isn't there. Since low blood sugar also "isn't there," the patient with elevated blood insulin—which can seriously disturb the brain and central nervous system—will be told that he has "imaginary hypoglycemia," although the treatment that controls hypoglycemia also controls the effects of excessive insulin levels: a corrected diet.

which the initial rise may not be satisfactorily high and the level remains low and constant for an extended period of time and then ultimately drops. This curve is found frequently in individuals whose life-style is boring, whose work is without challenge, and who find no satisfaction in themselves and their performance. In short, a flat response to a flat existence. It is as if the emotional brain were saying something like: "If you won't change what is boring me, I'll order the autonomic center to drop your sugar so low that the thinking brain won't be able to function, and maybe then you'll do something about the problem." For such patients, the diet alone isn't enough; there must be psychotherapy to help them to find satisfactions in their life-style and work, or strength and will to change them. With the diet alone as their treatment, such patients improve for six weeks and then are likely to recapture their symptoms in the original intensity. Where the hypoglycemic with the classic curve in the sugar test is likely to be restless, those with the flat curve tend to be zestless.

Before we discuss the diets used for hypoglycemia, there are some important points about the treatments other than diet, with which you should be reasonably familiar. When the pancreas is producing too much insulin, the body orders the adrenal glands to compensate by production of hormones which raise the blood sugar. This effort to offset the constant lowering of the sugar level by insulin constitutes a drain on the resources of the adrenal glands from which, ordinarily, they recover when the pancreas has been quieted by removing sugar and highly refined starches from the diet. In a small percentage of cases, the adrenal gland doesn't recover. In those, the physician may recommend a short course of adrenal-cortex injections, with the purpose of giving your own glands a rest by supplying what they normally produce. There are extremists who believe that all hypoglycemics need adrenal-cortex injections. I have recommended to physicians that they wait until the diet and supplements have been used for six weeks, for at that point a group of patients can be identified who have not responded satisfactorily, and these become candidates for the added help of the glandular injections.

The mention of supplements brings up another important point. I listed malnourishment as one of the forces which create hypoglycemia. Its impact is on the liver primarily, and contrary to the opinions of laymen and some physicianss, the liver is more fundamental in controlling sugar metabolism than the pancreas. This explains the use by some nutritionists of brewer's yeast and desiccated liver supplements to the hypoglycemic's diet. It is the liver which is targeted when these sources of high-quality protein and Vitamin B Complex are administered, for this organ is dependent on these nutrients. Multiple vitamin-mineral supplements are also used, for insurance in recovery from other deficiencies, and injections of vitamins—particularly the B Complex—may be instituted to speed the process. The injections solve another problem: long-continued malnourishment may impair digestive and absorptive efficiency, which in turn increases deficiency. Bypassing the digestive tract, via vitamin injections, breaks this vicious circle.

Following the lists of food families in the Appendix, you will find a typical hypoglycemia diet. It is but a sample, perhaps a starting point. Some people will need more carbohydrate than the sixty grams daily it supplies; some will not tolerate that much; all hypoglycemics will fare better when starches replace simple sugars. You will note that the diet suggests three small meals and three snacks daily. This pattern greatly improves the carbohydrate tolerance of hypoglycemics and, in one of the few generalizations possible in nutrition, it can be said that three larger meals daily, in place of the six, will retard the recovery of most sufferers with low blood sugar. The frequent small meals also help the body to manage cholesterol, and make weight control easier, too.

As I review what you have learned, it seems to me, and it may to you, that the task of helping your arthritis with good nutrition becomes progressively more difficult as you go from the no-nightshade diet to identification of allergies, and from there to control of hypoglycemia. Certainly, drug therapy is easier—if you are willing to accept symptomatic relief rather than full control of the disease and don't mind struggling with side reactions which sometimes are more threatening than the disorder being treated. Be of good cheer: not only is the game worth the candle, but as you read on, you will discover that we in nutrition have some very simple vitamin therapies for arthritis. One of them is the niacinamide treatment for osteoarthritis, developed and tested over many years by my friend Dr. William Kaufman, whose research I passingly mentioned earlier. Another is the Vitamin B_6–potassium therapy, for which Dr. John Ellis is best known.

Before we discuss those treatments, which like everything else we've discussed have been neglected in orthodox arthritis management, let me answer a question which may have occurred to you when I mentioned that the Appendix supplies a sample of a hypoglycemic diet: is there but one? Answer: there are a number of variations on the theme, and the choice should be made under the direction of a competent medical nutritionist. Another question: if hypoglycemia is fanning the flame of arthritis, how long should it take for the diet to produce results? As little as a week, but more commonly six weeks. Still another question: if one is an arthritic and a hypoglycemic, and the diet doesn't help the arthritis, is it worth staying on it? Answer: hypoglycemia is a multifaceted attack on well-being. Even if it is present, and relieving it doesn't relieve arthritic pains and aches in some degree—which ordinarily it would—there will be other dividends which you will find very rewarding, like a calmer nervous system, better sleep, better digestion, heightened resistance to infection, improved response to necessary medications, and—which usually happens—much more energy.

If you wish to know more about hypoglycemia, beyond the scope of this highlight discussion, I've already referred you to a book I devoted entirely to that subject. In another of my texts, * there is a series of letters from readers and listeners who had hypoglycemia which went undetected until they were fortunate enough to find the right physician. Their stories cover a spectrum from frustration, ill health, and defeat to heartwarming histories of recovery.

This journey through hypoglycemia would be incomplete if I omitted a commandment I must urge you to observe: learn to read food labels. If you don't, you'll never escape the sugar intake which is wrecking Americans, arthritic or not. Ingredients are listed on labels in the order of the percentages present, thus the first ingredient is the one of which there is the largest amount, the second is present in smaller amounts, and so on. Unfortunately, manufacturers who don't want you to realize how much sugar you're eating list sugars under different names. Thus sugar appears high on the list of ingredients, but corn syrup is listed later, and perhaps glucose, or honey, or fructose—and you don't realize that these are all sugar, and if the content of all forms of sugar were totaled, it might devolve that the ingredient which should lead the list, highest in percentage, is sugar! Few people realize that a doughnut has five teaspoonfuls of sugar, a glazed doughnut has seven, Shake 'n Bake is 50 percent sugar, ketchup is 23 percent, there is sugar in canned peas, and in salad dressings, and frankfurters, and—believe it or not—even in salt, when dextrose is added as an anticaking agent. If hypoglycemia is an entity in your pains, sugar is an entity in your troubles, and you must learn to avoid eating a teaspoonful of it every thirty-five minutes, twenty-four hours a day—which is the national average.

*Eat Well, Get Well, Stay Well (New York: Grosset & Dunlap, 1980, hardcover).

5

Rheumatoid Arthritis— The Price of Friendly Fire

Rheumatoid arthritis is one of a number of diseases in which the defense mechanisms of the body go strangely awry. In these, the immune system charged with defending the organism against bacteria, viruses, and cancer cells loses its ability to distinguish between the alien and the normal, and begins to attack the body itself. Hence the term "friendly fire," borrowed from the military description of casualties in our own troops as a result of misdirection of our own artillery or bomb attacks. No one knows what deceives the immune system into attacking its host, and thereby no one really understands how nutritional treatments may slow, stop, or sometimes reverse the process. That they must is obvious from the responses which sometimes occur to nutritional therapies in rheumatoid arthritis and other "autoimmune" disorders, though the orthodoxy would dismiss such recoveries as "spontaneous remissions"—improvements purely coincidental and owing nothing to the treatment. Though spontaneous recoveries from cancer are astronomically rare, I once heard an orthodox cancer specialist, watching one hundred terminal cancer patients respond to an unorthodox treatment, attribute *all* the recoveries to "spontaneous remission"!

When you've been exposed to infectious hepatitis, your physician may raise your resistance with an injection of gamma globulin. This use of a blood factor which is a normal constituent of the body's immune system would be your second experience, ordinarily, with medical augmentation of the body's own defenses, the first being your inoculations against measles, diphtheria, and other childhood infections. The current (and, I am convinced, unwarranted) excitement about interferon, a factor in cellular immunity, as a treatment for cancer is another example of the physician's increasing awareness of the untapped potential of the body's natural powers of resistance. As this research broadens, medical men will discover that the immune system is unbelievably sensitive both to the emotions and to nutrition. All this must come to pass before the constitutional, stressful, and nutritional forces which may trigger rheumatoid arthritis in the susceptible are fully understood, after which therapy will be based on that understanding, rather than on insensate overemphasis on palliative drugs with prohibitive side reactions and lack of genuine therapeutic effect.

In the preceding sentence, I listed three factors which affect the immune system, and which thereby should be considered in setting up treatment for rheumatoid arthritis (and other autoimmune diseases). The constitutional tendency does exist—I have read studies of body structure which indicate that children subject to rheumatic fever often display uniquely great differences in the structures of the two sides of the body. (Example: there is an average difference in the sizes of the right and left female breasts, but in these children, that is exaggerated to the point where one breast may be normal in size, and the other almost nonexistent.) The factor of the emotions operates as well: rheumatoid arthritics often have a poor sense of self-identity and a deep-seated dissatisfaction with their station in life. Indeed, the stress factor is explicitly recognized in the treatment of rheumatoids with hormones which are normally vital components of our antistress reactions. The factor of nutrition, though unexplored, is involved in many ways. One example is the stress which poor nutrition represents, both generically and in the failure of the diet to provide the nutrients, which support the antistress glandular functions. Not only have these forces remained unexamined as patients have been plied with aspirin and corticosteroids and gold, but in examining some common medical practices involving the immune system, one is almost driven to the conclusion that the profession, ignorantly if not advertently, was making a deliberate attack on it.

Take, for instance, the removal of tonsils, a type of surgery so common that it was sometimes performed in the physician's office, rather than in the hospital. In lieu of the surgery, radium "collars" were actually prescribed, bathing the tissues in constant irradiation, aimed at destroying the tonsils. How many cancers resulted from that procedure—which today would provoke suits for malpractice—is beside the point: the tonsil wasn't created to provide practice for surgeons. It is part of the body's immune system, painfully demonstrated by a higher incidence of a type of cancer (lymphoma) following tonsillectomies. We also came to realize that children minus tonsils had fewer sore throats but more bronchitis and pneumonia.

Today, with all this recognized, tonsils aren't removed unless they are grossly infected. But it is of more than academic interest to rheumatoid arthritics that tonsils are not only part of the immune system which in them has gone awry, but that the tonsils are sensitive to high intake of processed carbohydrates—of which many rheumatoid arthritics have consumed excessive quantities, often at the expense of adequate protein intake. There is, in fact, some evidence that pregnant women whose diet is high in refined carbohydrates may inflict enlarged tonsils and adenoids on the unborn. All this is of more than passing interest to the rheumatoid arthritic whose tolerance for sugars and starches is disturbed. It may explain why so many of these arthritics profit by a high protein diet, low in overprocessed starches and sugar.

The appendix, removal of which is the occasion for the most frequent emergency abdominal surgery in this country, has thus been the target for what turns out to be medical ignorance. Sometimes it was removed without reason other than the convenience offered by performance of other surgery in the abdominal area, which provided the opportunity to save the patient from a second operation to remove this "useless troublemaker." We now know that in some way, this organ, supposed to be an atavism, with no discernible function, is involved in the immune system. Some evidence has been provided, though ignored, by unaccustomed attacks of urticaria (hives) in patients recuperating from appendectomies. And ironically, we now have compelling evidence that appendicitis, rather than being a casual dispensation of a cruel fate, can be caused by lack of fiber in the diet, for the disease is extraordinarily rare in primitives whose intake of such bulkage is no more than three grams higher, per day, than ours.

Blundering medical attack on the thymus gland adds to the list of medical procedures which turned out to be unwitting assaults on the immune system. Irradiation of the thymus glands of infants was once widely practiced—on millions of babies—on the premise that the glands were abnormally enlarged and needed shrinking. But the "normal" size of the thymus was gauged by the size of the gland in adults, and years later it was recognized that the adults studied had died of wasting diseases which are known to shrink the thymus gland. Thus the babies' thymuses were not abnormally large, but had, tragically, been compared with abnormally small glands. "Tragically" because decades later, a large number of thyroid cancers were reported in those who had been subjected, as infants, to irradiation which spilled over to the throat area. More tragic, but as yet uninvestigated, is the strong possibility that diminishing the size of the thymus gland is actually a potent attack on the mainspring of the body's immune system. This would make us more subject not only to bacterial and viral infection, but also to cancer. It also raises a question to which there is again no answer: what's the possibility that disturbing the immune system invites rheumatoid arthritis (or other "autoimmune" diseases) in the susceptible? And how do you interpret the use of thymus hormones in cancer treatment?

As we have failed to realize the impact of surgery and irradiation on the body's defense system, so have we neglected the effects of food processing in depriving us of nutrients required by the immune mechanism. For example: there are reports in the medical literature that rheumatoid arthritics frequently have low levels of zinc in their hair and blood, and collateral studies which emphasize the improvements in the arthritis when zinc supplements are administered. Actually, these observations raise more questions than they answer. To begin, they pose a pointed question to our food industry: why do you persistently remove zinc from the carbohydrates from which we derive half our calories? To the Food and Drug Administration: why do you persistently create problems for the vitamin-mineral supplement industry, while viewing with equanimity and without criticism the removal of such nutrients from our food supply? And, apropos of other questions which are raised, we must ask whether the arthritic is benefiting by increased intake of zinc, or by the action of that metal in reducing elevated levels of copper which are common in rheumatoid arthritics. Any procedure which reduces abnormally high copper levels is beneficial, for elevation of copper is always harmful. But zinc is also a powerful stimulant to the immune system—so much so that even the orthodox literature in cancer research now cites that action. What's the chance that the zinc supplement helped the rheumatoid arthritics by correcting aberrations in the immune system?

We are left with the inescapable conclusion that the medical nutritionist must do what the orthodox rheumatologist bypasses: take a look at the zinc levels in rheumatoid arthritics, and raise them via zinc supplementing if needed. Physicians who don't want to subject patients to tests which insurance companies may not accept (and pay for) as necessary—though they don't object to bills for dangerous drugs —may go the other route: on the premise that a reasonable amount of zinc supplementing isn't going to cause trouble, they may routinely prescribe, say, fifty milligrams of zinc, in the form of zinc gluconate, daily, and observe the response. (P.S.: The insurance company may also refuse to pay for the zinc, though it will cheerfully pay for medication that relieves symptoms, presents toxicity, and doesn't correct the fundamental problems. Did you realize that the insurance carriers play a potent part in denying you the benefits of harmless treatments, on the grounds that they're "too innovative"?)

Very few physicians and medical or lay nutritionists appear to be aware of the importance of manganese to the thymus gland, though it was recognized years ago that atrophy can be traced to deficiency in this nutrient. In both animals and human beings, the thymus gland has been reported to recover from atrophy when manganese was administered. This observation was put to use years ago in the treatment of myasthenia gravis. It has not been applied as it should to rheumatoid arthritis. In any autoimmune disease, we are obligated to learn how to stimulate the immune system, or how to readjust the proportions of its many constituents when they aren't normal. Very few nutritional factors don't in some way affect that system favorably, including some—like zinc and Vitamin E—which are routinely removed from the processed sugars and starches which dominate our diets. I write that with emphasis gained from watching the gratifying responses in rheumatoid arthritics who were weaned away from processed carbohydrates, fed increased intake of high-quality protein, and given supplements of such nutrients as the Vitamin B Complex, Vitamin C, bioflavonoids, mixed tocopherols (the Vitamin E Complex), and zinc and manganese, among other minerals. Iron supplements and high-iron diets, incidentally, can't be recommended indiscriminately for rheumatoid arthritics, some of whom are victims of an excessive iron load.

Few are the nutritional factors which don't in some way meet a need of the immune system, including some—like Vitamin E—which have been ignored. It is this knowledge which frustrates the nutritionist as he reads statements like that of the American Medical Association when it termed Vitamin E to be "a vitamin in search of a disease." It is more the vitamin in need of intelligent investigation which is unhampered by opinionated ignorance, and it is one which often benefits the arthritic, in some instances because of its action on the immune system, in others because it has a beneficial effect on the pituitary gland, which is part of the "antistress" mechanism which functions poorly in rheumatoid arthritics. That last statement, incidentally, invokes a nutritional chemistry unknown to most researchers who have studied the vitamin. Concerning it, there is an axiom I trust (because I originated it) which says that a nutrient needed for the formation of a gland is very probably needed for its maintenance. In that light, how do you regard the fact that a minor degree of Vitamin E deficiency in the pregnant rat will cause the birth of young with pituitary glands half completed, looking as if surgery had been performed on them?

Earlier I remarked that if I were a rheumatologist, no patient would leave my office without tests for hypoglycemia and allergies and a trial of the no-nightshade diet with appropriate follow-up—meaning prescription of a diet for low blood sugar, if present. I earlier mentioned niacinamide supplements, the story of which you'll find in the next chapter. We can now add Vitamin E to the list, as well as the list of supplements given in a preceding paragraph.

Of all the experiments with nutritional therapies in arthritis, the strangest (and possibly the most ignored) was that recorded by English physicians. Because rheumatoid arthritics are stress prone, and the adrenal glands are pivotal in resistance to stress, therapy with adrenal hormones, such as cortisone, captured medical attention for years—at least, until it became plain that these powerful drugs caused more problems than they solved. The English researchers, aware that pantothenic acid is required by and stimulates the function of the adrenal glands, decided to study the effects of that vitamin on rheumatoid arthritics. They learned that large doses were helpful, but they encountered what seemed to be an invisible ceiling on blood levels of the nutrient—that is, increasing the dose beyond a certain point yielded no rise in the vitamin concentration in the blood. Aware that royal jelly, the food bees create for queen bees, is extraordinarily concentrated in pantothenic acid, they conjectured on the possibility that this food contains a factor or factors that might make the vitamin more effective. So it proved: royal jelly, given with the vitamin, removed the "invisible ceiling," and blood levels of pantothenic acid went up in proportion to increased dosages. As the blood concentration rose, benefits to the patients were similarly increased, though, of course, diminishing returns ultimately set in.

This research with pantothenic acid as a stimulant to adrenal function was not the only medical proof of that action. Esther Tuttle, M.D., years ago, demonstrated that the body's response to significant stress could be improved with high doses of pantothenic acid. Her subjects were butchers whose work took them alternately into walk-in freezers, with subzero temperatures, and then into rooms at normal temperatures. In response to this stress, their bodies reacted with increased levels of a type of cell called "eosinophils." Those levels were reduced when the men were given the vitamin. All this goes back to more basic studies by Dr. Agnes Faye Morgan, who was the first to demonstrate that deficiency in pantothenic acid causes degeneration of adrenal gland tissues, with internal bleeding and, interestingly, premature gray hair in animals. Restoration of the vitamin to the diet caused repair of the glands and recolored the hair.

Observations like these tend to drop into the well of yesterday's seven thousand years, rather than being picked up and acted upon by the medical establishment. The problem goes beyond medical apathy to the potential of nutrition as a force in prevention and treatment of disease. It also involves a strange tendency of physicians to regard glands as functioning autonomously, as if manufacturing their hormones out of the blue. The diet is, of course, the source of hormone precursors, and between nutrients and hormones there is a state of co- and counterplay, the effects so inextricably mixed that a deficiency of a nutrient may be displayed only as an imbalance of the glands, and vice versa. All this explains why research with pantothenic acid fell on deaf ears in the field of arthritis, which it did, for to this day, I don't recall a single paper recording any further study of the benefits this harmless vitamin might yield for rheumatoid arthritics. I do recall one adverse report: my good friend Dr. Carl C. Pfeiffer, of the Brain Bio Center notes that large doses of pantothenic acid caused minor erosions in the teeth to become more painful and joints more sore in arthritics. Certainly, Dr. Pfeiffer's observations demand attention. With equal certainty, I can say that this can't be a characteristic of all rheumatoid arthritics, for there are those who have benefited by the vitamin therapy without these side reactions, but I call it to your attention on the chance that you are such a reactor. If you are, the Pfeiffer group would restrict your pantothenic acid dose to thirty milligrams daily. This is far below the amounts used in the British research with the vitamin and royal jelly, in which such side reactions weren't reported.

It has been recorded that the white man, threatened with death by scurvy when snowed in, in northern Canada, has been rescued by native Indians, whose folklore taught them that the disease could be prevented or cured by eating the adrenal glands of deer. This primitive recognition of the fact that Vitamin C is concentrated in the adrenal glands has been confirmed by modern nutrition research, and from it we have learned that the content of the glands in the vitamin is depleted within minutes after the body is subjected to great stress. Exactly what role the vitamin plays in the chemistry of the glands, and how it assists the adrenals in resisting stress, no one understands, but there the fact is. Moreover, where depletion of the vitamin is rapid, restoration takes much more time. One wonders why, and one possible answer—assuming that the vitamin is in fact necessary to the antistress role of the adrenal glands—is that slow restoration is related to the fact that our Vitamin C requirements have been grossly underestimated. I am inclined to think so. Dr. Linus Pauling tells me that man, if able to synthesize the vitamin (which he can't), would on the basis of his body weight as compared with that of the creatures which do manufacture the vitamin, synthesize somewhere in the neighborhood of 2,200 milligrams daily. (The RDA—recommended dietary allowance—recently was *lowered* to 45 milligrams! This on the basis of the fatuous belief that the only function of the vitamin is prevention of scurvy.) Dr. Pauling estimates *normal* requirements for Vitamin C to be somewhere between 250 and 2,300 milligrams per day A rheumatoid arthritic, certainly not normal, could obviously need more. Particularly when his adrenal dysfunction is part of his disease, the vitamin is essential to the gland, and the aspirin he takes lowers blood levels of the vitamin. I have sometimes compromised, in setting up nutrition regimes for rheumatoid arthritis, by suggesting that the physician recommend the extended-release Vitamin C tablets previously mentioned, which allow generous blood levels to be maintained on, say, morning and evening doses of a 500-milligram sustained-release product.

The discovery of aspirin goes back ultimately to the belief of an English physician that Nature places remedies where she sites causes of disease. Rheumatic disorders tend to be more frequent in damp areas, like marshes, where grow the willow trees from which salicylic acid, the ancestor of aspirin, was isolated. It seems more than a pity that evidence which has a firmer basis in fighting rheumatoid disorders has been ignored. I have reference to repeated observations that children with rheumatic fever too often have a history of diets low in efficient protein—particularly, low in eggs. This folklore was investigated some years ago by the medical profession, in research involving two groups of children with rheumatic fever. Those with a severe form of the disorder were given two eggs daily, over and above any they had previously eaten. The other group were given the orthodox treatment: penicillin by mouth or by injection. At the end of the experimental period, the children fed the eggs had improved so much that their cases were then relatively the less serious; those on the antibiotic showed much less progress. (I often think of this experiment when I encounter the fanatic anticholesterol, antiegg theorists.) Question: was the lesson learned with the egg experiment ever put to use to help rheumatic fever? Was it ever applied to rheumatoid arthritics? Not to my knowledge, except in isolated instances where nutritionists, medical or lay, came to appreciate the specific importance of high-quality protein (eggs are the *highest*) in these illnesses.

You are entitled to ask at this point: have nutritionists like me seen all these data applied successfully in helping rheumatoid arthritics? Of course we have. That's one of the reasons for the writing of this book. I do want to make it exquisitely plain that the nutritional therapies for rheumatoid arthritis aren't panaceas. If, for instance, you bring your disease under control with applied nutrition, you will still be an easy target for stress—more so than the average person. If the stress becomes too great, it will climb over any nutritional wall we build, however stout, however high. And if you run into *two* significant stresses simultaneously, it will take more than nutrition to rescue you, for we are built to manage only one at a time.

A case history comes to mind, as I reread what I've just written. She is a young woman, mother of two, and one of my university students. She came to the courses in an effort to gain a background in nutrition, to let her escape the orthodox "treatment"—cortisone and aspirin—which her physician had forced upon her. When she announced that she was going to study nutrition, as a weapon against her disease, her medical man called her husband and said that he would not take the responsibility for the consequences if she discarded the drugs he had prescribed. In a year of formal study of nutrition—obviously, a course free of the dogmas of the hidebound dietician—she learned enough to bring her disease under satisfactory control. And by "control," I mean that she was well enough to go to work as an unpaid volunteer at a health center where modern nutrition is part of the resources drawn upon. The story of triumph has one flaw: one of her children developed a very serious disease for which there is no satisfactory treatment, and under the unbearable stresses associated with that, she suffered a relapse. It illustrates what I mean when I write that nothing builds a wall so high that stress can't climb it. When she resumed therapeutic, rather than maintenance, doses of the nutritional regime, and learned to cope with the problems presented by her son's illness, she responded again, and returned to work. All this, of course, was denominated as "spontaneous remission" by her cortisone-aspirin—minded physician.

As you will discover when you read chapter 6, niacinamide and other B vitamins have been used very successfully in the treatment of osteoarthritis. This, described as a "wear-and-tear" disease, in no way resembles rheumatoid arthritis, yet niacinamide therapy is used for both. The contradiction disappears when you realize that there is nothing to stop an unfortunate from having both diseases at once.

Osteoarthritis, as you might expect from its description as a wear-and-tear disorder, is obviously more common in older people, whereas rheumatic fever and rheumatoid arthritis can strike from childhood on, but there are age groups where the two types of arthritis can and do coexist. Thus large doses of niacinamide have been used to improve joint function in rheumatoids whose troubles are aggravated with stress at the joints over a long period of time. Please note that it isn't time alone that does it: I remind you again that there are arthritic children and healthy eighty-year-olds, and that the calendar doesn't cause arthritis. Since the factors of the Vitamin B Complex are important both to the immune system and to resistance to stress, as well as in carbohydrate metabolism, rheumatoid arthritics usually profit significantly by a supplement of these vitamins. If they also have osteoarthritis, the intake of niacinamide, as part of the Vitamin B Complex, is greatly raised, doses running into thousands of milligrams daily for some cases, as you will later read.

Many arthritics who have profited to any extent by drug therapy, without forbidding side reactions, are attracted to the possibility of added dividends from nutrition treatment, but concerned lest it interfere with the actions of the drugs. Such interference is rare to the point of improbability. If anything, the undesirable effects go in the opposite direction: the patient treated with corticosteroids and aspirin requires higher intake of nutrients to offset undesirable effects of the drugs. If anything, the interaction between nutrients and drugs enhances responses to the medications, reducing the doses needed and thereby lessening the likelihood and the severity of side reactions. Often drug doses can be lowered by significant amounts, and sometimes they can be entirely eliminated. I can think of only a few head-on collisions between nutritional and drug therapies. It isn't advisable to take iron medications when one is taking Vitamin E, or the doses should be separated by at least eight hours. It isn't intelligent to take estrogenic (female) hormone when one is being treated with Vitamin E, which is essentially an anti-estrogen factor, though it replaces the desirable effects of the dangerous hormone. Drug therapies and the no-nightshade diet, according to Dr. Childers, are an unhappy marriage, for nothing is gained and the benefits of the diet lessened or eliminated. Dr. Childers advises a gradual withdrawal of medication, under the physician's supervision, rather than sudden stopping for those for whom the diet proves helpful. When one is taking sulfa drugs PABA can't be used, for this type of antibiotic works by depriving bacteria of the PABA they need.

Beyond these examples, there is only one principle to remember concerning simultaneous use of medication with nutritional treatment: it's obvious that a well-fed person responds to *any* helpful therapy better than the poorly fed, and should and usually does require smaller doses of drugs, if any at all. That principle holds also for nondrug therapies, for physiotherapy, chiropractic, and osteopathic manipulation are essentially techniques of *mobilizing* the body's resources in battling disease and dysfunction; nutrition is a means of *increasing* those resources. From what you offer nutritionally, the body will make its selections on the basis of its inner wisdom—in a degree which passes belief. I have seen evidence that application of Vitamin E ointment to a normal muscle is followed in minutes by transfer of the vitamin to an adjacent muscle which is in spasm. Which reminds me: years ago, a physician reported that application of wheat germ oil ointment was markedly soothing to sore, spastic muscles. That report, too, has been ignored, although the treatment is harmless and sometimes surprisingly effective. Not only did the professions pass it by, but so did the vitamin industry, for I find that the few products which offer wheat germ oil in ointment form don't supply enough Vitamin E, and the Vitamin E ointments don't contain enough wheat germ oil. I bypass that problem by opening high-potency mixed tocopherol capsules, and squeezing the contents into any good wheat germ oil ointment, then mixing thoroughly. This has been a useful adjunct treatment for myositis, fibrositis, and other painful disorders. My data for the medical profession suggest that the patient be instructed to use the ointments without massage, since improperly done massage is worse than none at all, and the local application of the ointment is frequently helpful on its own. Some physicians have their patients apply the ointment and then cover the area with warm, moist towels or with an electric heating pad set at lowest temperature.

As I open a discussion of the diet—rather than individual nutrients—in the management of rheumatoid arthritis, there is an ancient and feeble joke which perfectly illustrates my professional problem. It is the story of a self-taught fiddler who sawed away at one single note on one single string. Other players change notes and utilize all strings, his tortured audience pointed out. His response was: "They're searching for their note. I found mine." There are many one-note players in nutrition. There are the incompetents who are convinced that good foods quarrel with each other, and can't be served at the same meal. There are the obsessed, who find the highest good in pure vegetarianism. There are the antifat, anticholesterol fanatics who must ignore a mountain of evidence to maintain their position. There are the competent who have become persuaded that a diet high in fish and brown rice and vegetables will prevent or reverse *all* arthritis. They all share the fundamental weakness of the fluoridation fanatics who would wipe out tooth decay by uniform addition of fluoride to drinking water which is consumed in differing quantities by people whose biochemistries are not uniform.

It would make life easier—at least for this nutritionist—to join the one-note players. It would also be a disservice to you. The effect of an insult is determined by the soil on which it falls. What constitutes an insult is defined by the target. There are those who thrive on vegetarian diets, and arthritics who profit by them. There are those who need the high quality of animal protein, and pay a bitter price if they lean on the weak straw of vegetable sources. There are those who gain health dividends from high intake of unprocessed carbohydrate, just as there are ulcer patients who would find such a diet an invitation to fresh attacks. Pointing out such individual differences earns the nutritionist no Brownie points. The public demands assured answers, not questions they've never considered. If you're of that persuasion, let me remind you that, like it or not, this book has strongly advised you to consider that your arthritis may involve three factors of individual differences in reaction to foods well tolerated by others: allergies, intolerances and hypoglycemia. But our differences go beyond allergies and intolerances, and I'll ask you to bear with me as I remind you that you are a unique event in the universe—and that applies even if you're one of a pair of "identical" twins.

I gave thiamin (Vitamin B_1) to a woman whose entire adult life had been spent as a recluse because of her stammering, which was so severe that she resorted to written notes to avoid conversation. She takes 100 milligrams daily, and so long as she does, her speech is fluent. A 2-milligram dose, which failed for her, was effective for another stammerer, and no amount helped the next four with whom I worked. High intake of choline, inositol, the Vitamin B Complex, and Vitamin E resulted in the disappearance of uterine fibroid tumors in a thirty-year-old woman. Her physician, in a subsequent operation, found, to quote his amazed comment, "vestigial buds." He had never seen that response. There were cases before her which didn't respond, and there will be successes and failures in the future. That applies to cystic mastitis, too. I know the chemistry involved; I don't know what happens to it in the failures. I do know people differ, and that is the point I want to emphasize before we discuss the diet in rheumatoid arthritis. Beyond considering acute individual differences like allergies or hypoglycemia, there are others with which we must reckon.

It isn't only the biochemical, neurological, or glandular

variation with which we must deal. Body structure is a variable which cloaks other differences. A disease—arthritis or whatever—will be more severe in a short person or a very tall person. Gall bladder syndrome is more common in women, and when it occurs in men they are likely to have certain feminine characteristics in their body build. Body structures conducive to stomach ulcer differ from those associated with duodenal ulcer, though the lesions are only a couple of inches apart. We are different.

If the statement still needs emphasis, consider that your body will reject a transplanted organ from your brother or your sister or your mother. It is alien tissue, that transplant, though from someone whose genes overlap yours. Individual, too, are those (few) human nutritional requirements which have been closely studied. Some people maintain calcium equilibrium with a quarter of a gram of calcium in the daily diet. Some need four times as much to reach the same balance. (This is one of the considerations behind formulation of a diet for an arthritic, for some of these patients tend to develop osteoporosis—weakening of the bones.) Protein requirements may vary by a factor of 6. Fat tolerances vary tremendously, and some people tolerate vegetable better than animal fats.

Perhaps the quickest way for you to appreciate the state of the art (nutrition) as applied to human beings derives from a symposium by the National Aeronautics and Space Administration, at which leading nutritionists were asked to set the menus for space flights of long duration. The agenda included requirements for protein, fat, carbohydrate, water, fiber, vitamin, minerals, and, of course, calories. The symposium disbanded without decisions. They couldn't even arrive at a consensus on calories. And this was a failure in dealing with meals for a captive group—isolated in a space ship—all in superb health. How can anyone inflict uniform dietary recommendations on people who are not in superb health, who are sick, who are not captive but capable of evading dietary dictates, and who are biochemically unique? And whose uniqueness may include aberrations of body chemistry like allergy, hypoglycemia, diabetes, and other metabolic disorders?

You have just read my reasons for rejecting the sweeping generalizations behind the high-carbohydrate, high-vegetable, high-anything diets. And if you accept what I've reviewed for you—and you really have no choice—then you know that I can't follow this discussion with a series of menus. Let me give you the generalizations which are possible and assign to you—on the basis of enlightened consent and cooperation—the task of working out your nutritional destiny.

To establish the boundaries of your personal needs and tolerances in diet for arthritis, what you have read dictates these steps:

1. Elimination of the nightshades from your diet. This can be done on a pure trial-and-error basis, or you can try the simple kinesiological test for intolerance to peppers, white potato, eggplant, tomato, and tobacco. Remember that *all* members of the pepper family are nightshades, except black and white pepper.

2. If you are intolerant of the nightshades, you must compensate for the nutrients you will sacrifice by avoiding these foods. These are principally vegetable Vitamin A (carotene) and Vitamin C. The white potato also supplies a small amount of Vitamin B_6. Dark-green vegetables and carrots will replace the nightshades effectively as sources of carotene. Fruits will supply Vitamin C, of course, with citrus particularly recommended if you tolerate them, for they also yield the bioflavonoids. Animal proteins (meat, fish, fowl, eggs, cheese, and milk products) will

yield Vitamin B_6, as will whole grains, brewer's yeast, wheat germ, and bran.

3. It's obvious from what you've read that you *must*, by the most convenient and efficient methods available to you, exclude from your diet any foods to which you are allergic. Once you've identified such allergies, be sure to look up the food families in the Appendix, to guide yourself away from the related foods.

4. If the list of foods forbidden by allergy is lengthy enough to make menus difficult to assemble while preserving good nutrition, consult one of the recommended texts to learn how to manage the four-day rotation diet. If that proves difficult, consult a bioecological allergist or a medical nutritionist for supervision.

5. Check your symptoms against the home test for low blood sugar, given in chapter 4. If your score is 58 or over, use the visit to the medical nutritionist or bioecological allergist for the medical test for hypoglycemia. If your score is high enough, the physician may choose to place you on the hypoglycemia diet as a "therapeutic diagnosis." Translation: if your symptoms lessen or disappear while you're on the diet, the response confirms it: you had hypoglycemia.

6. If you do have the glucose tolerance test, and it does indicate hypoglycemia, you may find that the diet improves your health and lessens your symptoms, but not enough; or you may show no response at all. If you encounter either of these eventualities after six weeks on the diet, your physician may recheck you for allergies to the foods the diet permits. There are two possibilities: some of those allergies may have been missed in your earlier testing, or you may have

developed some new ones. Another possibility: you show improvement on the diet during the first six weeks, and it may be quite significant, but then improvement slows down. It is as if you had reached a threshold you can't penetrate. At this point, your doctor may decide that your adrenal glands are weary from years of trying to offset your low blood sugar, and give them a rest by injecting adrenal cortex hormones. Such injections for the small percentage of patients who need them often have a startling effect on well-being and energy, and are frequently effective in overcoming residual impotence in the male or frigidity in the hypoglycemic female.

7. When it is a rheumatoid arthritic who is hypoglycemic, it will be understandable, from what you have read, if the physician insists that you consume two or three eggs daily, as part of the protein in the diet. Contrary to what you have read, in individuals whose blood fats are within normal range, an intake of *thirty-five* egg yolks daily has been reported to cause no significant change in blood cholesterol. This observation was made by Israeli physicians, feeding tremendous amounts of eggs to help provide the high-quality protein needed for healing of burns. The medical nutritionist will, of course, have checked your blood chemistry as a background for his recommendations.

8. The supplements listed in this chapter are used at two different levels of dosage. The lower level is that used to assure adequacy of intake. It offsets losses of vitamins in processing, storage, and cooking and compensates for poor absorption. It also is helpful to those with elevated re-

quirements which are difficult to satisfy from food alone, without running the risk of unwanted weight gain. The second level of dosage is much higher. Its purposes overlap those of the lower level, but add therapeutic action. To be sure you understand the distinction, consider a supplement of twenty-five milligrams of zinc daily. This is the lower level, and protects you against inadequacy of zinc intake. Against this is the quantity the physician might prescribe if he finds that you, like other rheumatoid arthritics, have elevated copper levels in the blood. He might prescribe the same amount three times daily, or even more.

I am giving you these details so that you understand that I don't want to encourage self-medication, but I do want to be sure that your diet supplies what you need for decent health. At the lower level, I want the diet in rheumatoid arthritis supplemented with cod-liver oil, Vitamin C, bioflavonoids, zinc, Vitamin E (mixed tocopherols), and manganese. Many of these factors are available combined in a single tablet or capsule, with dosages ranging from one or two up to six or eight capsules daily. I prefer the supplements of natural origin—not because there is any discernible difference between a natural vitamin and its synthetic duplicate, but because there are trace amounts of other nutrients in the natural sources and, even more importantly, because the manufacturers of natural supplements are likely to avoid the added sugar, starch, preservatives, coal-tar dyes, and other additives frequently found in synthetic vitamin supplements.

Brewer's yeast, wheat germ, and desiccated liver are useful natural sources of the unknown factors in nutrition, but allergy to these foods, which contain hundreds of factors, is of course possible, as is allergy to the vitamins, and it is important to be sure that none of these supplements evokes intolerance or allergic reactions.

In the Appendix, I have listed levels of supplementary intake of the nutrients we have discussed. There are two vitamins which need detailed study and which we have not yet discussed. These are niacinamide and pyridoxin (Vitamin B_6). As you will discover, physicians have been using tremendous doses of these factors in osteoarthritis. The pioneering research was performed by Dr. John Ellis, with Vitamin B_6, and Dr. William Kaufman, with niacinamide and, frequently, added amounts of other B vitamins. In the discussions of these therapies, we shall be dealing with doses astronomically beyond the amounts ordinarily incorporated in daily vitamin supplements. By use of these therapies, the two physicians achieved reputations for rescuing thousands of patients from the agonies of arthritis, and their stories are well worth reading.

6

"You Rescued Me from the Prison of Arthritis"

I took my undergraduate work at the University of Alabama, not far from the Hillman Clinic, where Dr. Tom Spies conducted his pioneering research in the prevention and treatment of pellagra. His findings confirmed those of earlier investigators who had blamed this disease on a diet low in protein and the B Complex vitamin, niacinamide. Oddly, Dr. Abram Hoffer's successful use of niacinamide in the treatment of early schizophrenia derived almost directly from Dr. Spies' use of the vitamin for the treatment of pellagra, an unrelated disease; and still more oddly, Dr. William Kaufman's use of niacinamide in the treatment of osteoarthritis was also inspired by Spies' findings. Dr. Hoffer was intrigued by the pellagrins who hear imaginary voices, which some schizophrenics do too; and Dr. Kaufman was impressed by the disappearance of joint pains in pellagrins treated with niacinamide. The parallel goes beyond these points, for Hoffer has written a poignant description of his aged mother's response to large doses of niacinamide for her arthritis (and other symptoms usually considered to be the price of senility), and Kaufman, while primarily interested in the response of arthritics to doses of the vitamin, noted that it slows or reverses many symptoms which are ordinarily blamed on aging.

The paths of the two pioneers crossed when Dr. Hoffer was given credit for initiating the use of "megavitamin" doses of niacinamide in schizophrenia, and Dr. Kaufman wrote to him to claim the priority every man of science treasures, pointing out that his use of large doses of the vitamin preceded Hoffer's by a number of years. I already knew Dr. Hoffer, having gone to Canada to observe his application of orthomolecular treatment in schizophrenia, and this was the trail I followed which enabled me to meet Dr. Kaufman. After examining his papers and other publications on niacinamide therapy for osteoarthritis, I was so impressed with his research, and so furious with the arthritis establishment for ignoring it for more than twenty years, that I proposed for him the honor of delivering the annual Tom Spies Memorial Lecture at the annual convention of the International Academy of Preventive Medicine, of which I have been an officer. The Academy found Dr. Kaufman's credentials and research impressive, and what you are about to read is the lesson in nutrition versus arthritis which he taught to the hundreds of physicians who heard his paper read.

In detailing the responses of thousands of arthritics to niacinamide and other vitamin therapies, Dr. Kaufman emphasized that his observations did not rest on subjective reports from his patients—that is, on symptomatic relief which only the patient could detect. This physician also has a Ph.D. degree in physiology, and used that expertise to develop objective measurements of the progress of the vitamin-treated patients. In these he included impaired joint mobility, impaired muscle strength, reduced maximal muscle working capacity, impaired sense of balance, and "certain geriatric mental syndromes." It is important for you to realize that some of these responses included disabilities frequently charged to the aging process itself, rather than to arthritis alone.

Though the process of measuring objective responses to the vitamin treatment consumed from three to five hours for the initial visit to the doctor's office, and one to two hours for subsequent checkup visits, the young physician

113

persisted, painstakingly recording for each patient:

> Verbatim records of everything said during an office visit.
>
> Biomicroscopic examinations of the soft tissues—the external surfaces of the eyes and inner surfaces of the lids—lips, gums, tongue, and skin.
>
> All this was also recorded in color pictures. In female patients, he also examined and color-photographed the cervix.

To these records, he shortly added measurements of the patients' "joint range index." If you fold your fingers so that the tips are touching the palm, as close as possible to the base of the fingers, you have an idea of what is meant by the joint range index, which in arthritics, obviously, is usually impaired. Using a simple mechanical device, the young doctor measured the patient's strength and maximal working capacity. As part of the troubles of these vitamin-deficient arthritics, Dr. Kaufman found that their sense of balance was frequently disturbed, though many of them were unaware of that before it was tested. In some cases, he warned those hearing his paper, physicians would have to be cautious in testing the balance sense, for some of the patients, if not closely watched, could have a serious fall.

Significantly, Kaufman found it helpful to use the food-symptom diary which I have recommended to you. The diary not only made it possible for him to monitor the adequacy of the patients' menus, but also helped in tracking down food-related allergic and psychosomatic reactions, all of which contributed to their debilitation.

The physician who is "the new kid on the block" is very likely to attract the patients who haven't been helped by other physicians and other treatments. They come to the doctor without hope, in despair about their health problems. So Dr. Kaufman describes his first seven patients, to whom he credits his shift from cardiology, which was his first love in medicine, to the study and treatment of diseases caused by poor nutrition.

Dr. Kaufman's research in the effects of niacinamide deficiency began several years before enrichment of bread and intake of multiple vitamin supplements raised the niacinamide intake of the public. When it did, the symptoms changed.

Before niacinamide levels were raised, Dr. Kaufman observed in his patients—both the arthritic and the nonarthritic —anxiety, depression, personality changes, excessive startle reaction to noise, excessive fear of physical injury, impaired sense of balance, numbness, tingling, and other sensory disturbances. Skin symptoms were frequent, as were digestive disorders, and there were adverse changes in the tissues of the mouth and in the muscles controlling the tongue. Impairment of both muscle strength and maximal muscle working capacity were frequent, as were reduction of joint mobility and sensitivity of cartilage to pressure from a finger. All these and other components of the niacinamide-deficiency syndrome were relieved when the vitamin was given, and returned when the patient stopped the treatment and returned to a usual diet.

In these responses, Dr. Kaufman saw the essential difference between orthodox medicine and what is now called "holistic medicine." His own words are striking, but the language is technical, and I should like to paraphrase what he said, for it is as much a commentary on fragmented treatment of arthritis as it is a comparison of traditional with avant-garde medicine.

Here is a patient, the doctor reminded his audience, with symptoms which I knew to be caused by dietary deficiency. Questions:

> Should the anxiety be treated with a tranquilizer? Should the depression be treated with an antidepressant?

Should the digestive disturbances be medicated with atropine?

Should I recommend ointments to soften the calluses?

Should douches be prescribed for the inflammation of the vaginal tissues?

Should diuretics be used to drive the water out of the swollen tissues?

Should aspirin or related drugs be recommended to reduce the discomfort of the bones and joints?

Dryly, the physician said that he gave due consideration to all these options—acceptable to any orthodox physician—and decided that all the symptoms came from a single cause: lack of adequate amounts of niacinamide in all the cells of the patient. As the logical consequence, he bypassed all the drugs and used niacinamide as the only therapeutic agent.

At the time when Dr. Kaufman was treating his early patients, he used what he then considered to be adequate—but now realizes to be low—doses of niacinamide, ranging from fifty to one hundred milligrams, three times daily. The responses were fast and great enough, as he put it, to jar his sense of reality. He describes what happened with a single dose, by mouth, of one hundred milligrams of niacinamide, administered to the patient with the doctor observing. Swelling of the tissues began to reduce in ten to fifteen minutes. At that time, there was measurable improvement in the strength of the muscles and in maximal muscle working capacity in many patients (though not all). The disturbance in the sense of balance sometimes receded within thirty to sixty minutes after the dose of niacinamide, although weeks to months of treatment with this vitamin (plus other B vitamins, on occasion) were sometimes necessary before the balance sense really reached normal. Within a few days of niacinamide treatment, the anxiety, depression, tingling, and digestive complaints disappeared. Usually in one or two weeks, but sometimes taking as long as two or three months, the tenderness and enlargement of the liver were not apparent to the examiner, and the vaginal redness and tenderness yielded within two to ten days of continuous therapy with niacinamide. Similar improvements showed in pigmentation of the skin, in tenderness of the cartilage, and in redness and swelling of the tongue, although some of the symptoms took but a week to improve and others as long as three months to several years.

The observation which was critical for arthritics was the joint range index. Even with doses of the vitamin that Dr. Kaufman now recognizes as low, he was able to observe measurable improvement in some of the joints in patients with hypertrophic or rheumatoid arthritis, and in other patients who had impairment of joint mobility with no external evidence of arthritis. Later, he came gradually to realize that larger doses of niacinamide were needed, and sometimes doses of other B vitamins, as well, although niacinamide remained his chief weapon in arthritis. He found that he had to raise the intake of niacinamide to somewhere between 1,500 and 4,000 milligrams daily, in divided doses. Only at such levels could he benefit the patient with the maximum improvement in joint mobility, and that response was based on several ifs"—If the niacinamide dose was adequate, if the patient's diet was adequate, particularly in protein and calories, if the joints were not being subjected to constant injury, and if none of the joints had been previously so damaged that recovery was impossible.

During the years of World War II, enrichment of bread with vitamins, including niacinamide, became compulsory. Dr. Kaufman saw the results of the increased vitamin intake in many patients in his practice. Many of the symptoms attributable to niacinamide deficiency became less severe, less common, or disappeared. These included anxiety, depression, excessive fear of being hurt, intestinal symptoms, tenderness of cartilage, and most of the other disturbances mentioned earlier in this chapter. But some of the symptoms didn't respond. These included the adverse changes in membranes in the mouth, reduction of muscle strength, lessened maximum muscle working capacity, impaired sense of balance, a mild depression or agitation in elderly people, and—which is important for the arthritic—impaired joint mobility.

The physician's interpretation of the persistence of some of the symptoms of niacinamide deficiency, even after bread enrichment had raised the public's intake of the vitamin, was logical. A nutritionist might have speculated on the easy possibility that people who are watching their calories tend to restrict their intake of bread, and thereby restrict their dividends from the vitamin enrichment. The medical man concluded that some tissues need far less additional niacinamide than others, to function at improved levels. The other side of the coin is obvious: the tissues that didn't profit by increased niacinamide intake from enriched bread obviously needed much more of the vitamin than the others did. He targeted those: tissues with a high niacinamide need included muscles, movable joints, tongue membrane, that section of the spinal cord important to the function of the sense of balance, and, in those over fifty-five, certain parts of the brain.

Let me translate what he is saying that is vital to an arthritic: it is possible to have a deficiency of niacinamide which doesn't cause the symptoms of pellagra, because the deficit of the vitamin isn't that great, but which *is* significant enough to cause muscular weakness, degeneration of movable joints, and disturbances of the sense of balance.

There are two notes I should like to add to that, derived from years of observation of the responses of patients to deficiency and to treatment. Not only are some tissues more susceptible to nutritional deficiency than others, but in each patient there is likely to be an "Achilles' heel"—which is simply to say that human brains are all dependent on an adequate supply of niacinamide, but my brain may react earlier and more violently than yours. Thus an inadequate intake of niacinamide might make me feel "swimmy-headed" (the actual phrase patients use to describe the effect), while in you, the very same degree of deficiency might strike at your joints, leaving the brain, at least for a while, unaffected. One of the determining factors other than constitutional differences may be the amount of demand one puts on the organ, system, or tissue—how much pressure there is on the brain and nervous system, how much stress is inflicted on the joints.

Since the problems of arthritics include muscle pain and easy muscle fatigue, it will be interesting for you to observe a young man, nonarthritic, whose complaint is primarily directed to his excessive fatigue when he exerts himself physically in any way. Tested for maximum muscle working capacity, he was 11 percent below the lower limit of normal, though he had no discomfort during the test. Only ten minutes after he has taken 100 milligrams of niacinamide, his muscle working capacity has improved measurably. In thirty minutes, it has risen 50 percent and holds that level for the next hour and a half. Dr. Kaufman points out that the early rise in his maximum working capacity exactly corresponds with rising levels of niacinamide in the blood, and with spontaneous comments from the patient to the effect that he is feeling better. This young man was dosed with 100 milligrams of niacinamide three times daily, and within a week, lost all his complaints of fatigue. The doctor points out that the twenty-four-year-old appeared healthy and athletic, but with his original complaints of easy fatigability he might—just because he appeared robust—have been labeled as a hypochondriac by physicians less aware of the impact of nutritional deficiencies.

With the next patient, Dr. Kaufman tells us of an older person—sixty—who also showed excessive fatigability and yet had high normal muscle strength. But she also displayed symptoms of niacinamide deficiency in the tongue membrane and in impaired sense of balance, muscle working capacity, and mobility of the joints. Given 300 milligrams of niacinamide every three hours, six doses daily, she responded with normal resistance to fatigue, significant improvement in the mobility of her joints, and lessening of her other symptoms, including the disturbed sense of balance. Dr. Kaufman places particular emphasis on the need for careful medical testing of the balance sense, particularly in older people, for he found it often disturbed, frequently without the patient's realizing it, and a sensitive index of the effects of niacinamide deficiency. Improvement in it, in muscle function, and in mobility of the joints is a recurring observation in the doctor's some thirty years of observations of the responses of arthritics to niacinamide therapy. It should be emphasized that other B vitamins were sometimes found useful and necessary in the treatment. The addition of thiamine and riboflavin made a significant difference to some patients whose muscle strength and working capacity had not responded to niacinamide alone. Other patients also received doses of choline, which proved particularly helpful for flabby muscles. In these cases, the patients developed muscle tone one would expect, the doctor notes, in persons doing heavy manual labor. (This action of choline isn't mysterious. I have capitalized upon it for years in such muscle disorders as myasthenia gravis, for the nutrient is essential to the manufacture of a chemical which mediates control of the muscles by the nervous system.)

Dr. Kaufman is claiming no panaceas, acknowledging that in 30 percent of the patients no type of vitamin treatment remedied muscular weakness, fatigability, impaired grip strength, or impaired muscle working capacity. It is probably not significant, but it is interesting that his percentage of failure is identical with that reported by Dr. Childers with the no-nightshade diet. I have already indicated my interest in seeing the two types of treatment combined. It would be logical, for the nightshade's toxic chemical, solinase, interferes with the neuromuscular chemistry which the vitamin therapy is intended to improve.

Repeated references to the patients' impaired sense of balance may be misleading, both to the layman and to the physician inexperienced with the effects of nutritional deficiency on this function. A difficulty in walking (ataxia) or uncertainty in the sense of balance have been observed in many patients with varying degrees of niacinamide deficiency. They usually don't complain of being dizzy or having an unjustified feeling of falling, but when they change position suddenly, they obviously lose their balance. They sometimes stagger in walking, and are subject thereby to severe bumps and dangerous falls. As every layman knows, tests of the balance sense are usually performed with the eyes closed. The person who fails that test—if aged—is particularly in danger when walking in the dark. Dr. Kaufman warns his fellow physicians that the conventional balance test (Romberg) isn't rigorous enough, and that more strenuous testing may be needed to elicit the symptoms in the patients with niacinamide deficiency. One is driven here to reflect that the practitioner who is not nutrition conscious may blame disturbances of the balance sense on aging itself, exactly as he describes arthritis, with its muscle pain and restricted joint mobility, in terms of "Of course you have arthritis—you're getting old."

All this preoccupation with the sense of balance may frustrate you a reader interested in arthritis. The discussion isn't pointless. Put simply: *if you have a niacinamide deficiency which is impairing your sense of balance, it may also be contributing to your muscle weakness and to your painful restriction of joint mobility.*

With sufficient dosage of niacinamide, many (but not all) patients recover normal sense of balance, which must eventuate within three months of the start of treatment, if it is to occur. Some people will need thiamine, B_6, and B_{12} in addition to niacinamide therapy. If the treatment is effective, stopping it will quickly demonstrate that the recovery isn't a triumph of faith healing. Dr. Kaufman is quick to note, though, that those who fail to achieve normal balance sense do benefit in other ways. These included correction of mild depression or agitation or restlessness in patients over fifty-five, many of whom, however, required the other vitamins in addition to niacinamide. All this, of course, illustrates the truth of the ancient nutritional maxim: nutritional deficiencies in man are likely to be multiple.

One would suppose that the physician would be satisfied with the benefits his vitamin research had brought to his patients. Certainly, they were great enough to persuade the medical man to switch from cardiology to nutrition in medicine. But these accomplishments, in his own eyes, pale before what he considers his most important contribution to nutritional medicine. He puts it in medical language, which I have translated for you:

Adequate treatment with niacinamide, added to a diet supplying enough protein and calories, can improve impaired mobility of the joints in persons of all ages, whether or not they have visible arthritic deformities. There are two qualifying provisos: obviously, the joints must not be so badly damaged that recovery isn't possible, and equally obviously, the joints must not be subjected to renewed, repetitive injury.

Kaufman's discovery that niacinamide had a beneficial effect on mobility of the joints was, like so many others of its type, an "astonishing" accident. He was treating the symptoms of pellagra, and never anticipated that "stiff joints would become more flexible." But they did. And that led the physiologist-physician to study very carefully the ranges of joint movement in all his patients prior to and during treatment with niacinamide. Among other striking observations, he came to realize that the mobility of the joints was affected twenty or more years *before* the obvious evidence of arthritis appeared, in the form of what the physicians call "Heberden's nodes." In fact, he emphasizes that many people who had no visible arthritic deformities suffered just as severe limitations of joint mobility, in certain aspects of motion, as those who visibly were suffering with osteoarthritis or rheumatoid arthritis. The importance of this observation invites us to pause to take a look at what is really happening to us.

In any average group of Americans, there are probability statistics applicable which, based upon experience in longevity and in the incidence of degenerative disease, allow us to make a prophecy for their futures. Thus I can say that at least 60 percent of the adults reading this book will live at least to the age of sixty-five. But 60 percent of those who survive will develop arthritis, diabetes, hypertension, heart disease, hardening of the arteries, kidney disease, or some other disabling, disagreeable, and life-shortening degenerative disorder. That means one in three of you (adults) who are reading these lines. Note that the list comprises the conditions for which medicine has few explanations and fewer remedies and, usually, no cures. That is what underlines the importance of Dr. Kaufman's observations that osteoarthritis, mislabeled as an inevitable concomitant of the aging process, begins years before there is any disability or abnormality which present medical examinations will recognize and, moreover, that there exists a vitamin therapy which may stop or reverse or control those degenerative changes in the joints, if they are not permitted to go to the point of no return. Compare this philosophy with that of the physicians who endlessly warn the public of vague (and undocumented) dangers of what they choose to call "excessive" vitamin intake.

By carefully analyzing all that he had learned from his studies of the responses of the joints of his niacinamide-treated patients, Dr. Kaufman was able to select twenty separate joint ranges which could be measured with facility, and which were likely to be the targets for the earliest impairment of joint mobility. The average of these joint measurements could be calculated, and became what he called the joint range index. (I give you all this detail so that you can see how carefully, how scientifically these studies of

Arthritis: Don't Learn to Live with It

niacinamide versus arthritis were conducted, and how unforgivable it is that the arthritis orthodoxy not only ignores the research, but discourages physicians from applying it.)

So sensitive is the joint range index that it not only tells the physician how much niacinamide the patient requires, but will reveal regression when the patient, without telling the doctor, reduces his dose of the vitamin, or takes it all at once instead of following the spacing of doses necessary to maintain the blood level of the vitamin.

After becoming acquainted with Dr. Kaufman's research, I reviewed it in several papers on arthritis, delivered at various medical societies of which I am a member, and found that both physicians and chiropractors tended to the conclusion—which is facile but unjustified—that niacinamide must have previously unsuspected pain-killing effects. An alternate theory had it that the vitamin must raise the patient's pain threshold, meaning that he becomes less sensitive to and less likely to perceive pain until it rises above an elevated level. Not so. Dr. Kaufman himself says emphatically that many patients have markedly lessened joint discomfort and pain as recovery progresses, but this does not mean that the vitamin is acting as a mere substitute for aspirin or codeine. Another reaction from my professional listeners involved the possibility that niacinamide has a hormone effect, like that of cortisone. Again, although it reduces inflammation as the corticosteroid hormones do, the vitamin is not acting as a hormone, however effectively it may (and often does) reduce inflammation. What it does do, among its many actions, is to favor the repair of the damaged surfaces common in degenerative or osteoarthritis. It acts as a tissue-building agent, in this sense, with a gentle action which is so slow that the doctor warns physicians that they must measure the joint mobility at each visit if they are to be aware of the significant improvement in the joints.

Repeatedly, the researcher warns that the vitamin treatment will be ineffective if the diet is low in calories or in

124

protein, and will be negated if the patient's occupation, for example, continues to inflict injury to the joints. While many joint surfaces are damaged to the point of no return, the physician emphasizes that it takes a long trial of niacinamide treatment to determine if this is so, for even severely damaged areas may recover in some degree.

Emphasis is great on the need not only to prescribe the right dose of niacinamide, but at the right intervals. The vitamin breaks down in the body in a relatively short time, and it is subject to excretion in the urine. For these reasons, frequency of doses is as important as the total amount taken daily; that is, a single dose of 1,500 milligrams of niacinamide, or three doses of 500 milligrams each, will not be effective in maintaining blood levels and vitamin activity if the required schedule is 250 milligrams to be taken every three hours, for six doses. The total is the same, but the action will be different. Based upon the joint range index—the average of twenty measurements of the performance of twenty joints—Dr. Kaufman carefully indicates not only total dosage, but the frequency of the smaller ones which make it up.

Considering a joint range index of 96–100 as normal, needing no treatment, the physician lists progressively more severe conditions with appropriate doses and frequency of doses of niacinamide:

86–95 (slight joint dysfunction): 900–1,500 milligrams of niacinamide daily, divided into six doses, taken every three hours.

71–85 (moderate joint dysfunction): 1,500–2,000 milligrams of niacinamide daily, divided into six doses, one every three hours, or eight doses, one every two hours.

56-70 (severe joint dysfunction): 2,000–2,500 milligrams daily, every two hours for eight doses, or every one and a half hours for ten doses.

55 or less (extremely severe joint dysfunction):
2,500 to 4,000 milligrams daily, divided into ten
doses, one every one and a half hours, or sixteen
doses, one every hour.

In a number of conversations with Dr. Kaufman, I came
to the erroneous conclusion that this vitamin therapy is applicable only to osteoarthritis. (That isn't a deprecating
statement: it's an accomplishment to benefit patients who
have been told they must take aspirin and learn to live with
the disease.) After studying his papers and monographs,
however, I realized that I was underestimating the treatment.
Kaufman notes that rheumatoid arthritis is much more complex than hypertrophic arthritis because of the allergic, im-
munologic, and glandular factors which enter into its causes,
but—a very important "but"—rheumatoid arthritis is always
superimposed on degenerative changes, in some degree, in
the cartilages at the joints, so that niacinamide is capable of
helping patients with either type of the disease.

One of Kaufman's case histories beautifully illustrates the
benefits of the vitamin therapy, the importance of the correct daily dose and the spacing of the smaller doses which
comprise it, and the influence of the patient's habits on recovery (or nonrecovery) from joint damage. The woman is
seventy-seven years old, which tells us that old age is not an
insuperable obstacle to the medical nutritionist. She has degenerative arthritis, on the edge of being extremely severe.
Her joint range index is 55.7. Until her fifth visit, her index
showed satisfactory improvement on her dose of 250 milligrams of niacinamide, taken every one and a half hours, for
ten doses a day. The patient decided to alter that schedule,
and took 500 milligrams, every three hours, in five doses
daily. The total daily dose was the same, but the benefits,
measured by the joint range index, were cut by 50 percent.
When she returned to the original schedule, she recaptured
her improvement, progressing from the lowest range of se-

vere joint dysfunction to about the middle range of moderate dysfunction.

Because of the multiple examinations of the mobility of twenty joints, to compile the joint range index, Kaufman is able to give us a beautifully detailed view of the progress of his patient. Hips, knees, and shoulders improved. The wrists responded the least because she constantly insulted those joints by holding tightly to bannisters as she pulled herself up the steps. Here, then, the battle was won by insults from the life-style, but overall, the niacinamide therapy significantly benefited her. And that sentence really hides more than it reveals in terms of the beneficial impact of niacinamide treatment on this woman's quality of life. Dr. Kaufman notes that she began treatment decrepit and depressed, unable to sit down unassisted in a chair, or leave it; unable unassisted to mount or leave a toilet seat, and requiring the help of a strong person even to enter or leave her bed. When she had been helped into a standing position, she had trouble remaining in it, difficulty in walking and keeping her balance, and thereby used two canes, which she clutched so tightly that her finger joints became painful. She could not comb her hair, she was bound to her chair and to her house, and, not unexpectedly, she wept frequently.

Three months of niacinamide treatment banished her depression and her crying. On her own, she could now sit down in a chair, and stand up, use a toilet, lie down in and rise from bed. She was able for the first time in many years to comb her hair. Some of her joints would never again be totally mobile, but her remarkable overall improvement was mirrored in a remark she made to her doctor on her last visit. Cheerful and spry and now physically active, the eighty-year old patient told the physician that she had been able to resume social and church activities. She kissed him on the cheek, and said: "You liberated me from the prison of my arthritis."

As I wrote the preceding lines, I was reminded of a leaflet

issued "as a public service" by the Health Education Center of Lenox Hill Hospital in New York City. It is titled "Information for People with Arthritis." The subtitle is "Quackery and Diet." Let me quote a few statements:

> Legitimate treatment for arthritis involves a regimen of: Medication—Special Exercise—Rest and all should be carried out under the close supervision of a qualified physician.
>
> Many people believe that special foods, or some exotic diet will prove helpful in relieving arthritis. This is not true. The possible relationship between diet and arthritis has been thoroughly and scientifically studied, and the fact is. . . *no food* has anything to do with causing arthritis and no food is effective in *treating* or "curing" it.
>
> Consult a qualified physician, and don't waste your money on the big business of food faddism.

The leaflet gives a clear-cut warning. Don't risk the benefits of a diet and vitamin therapy supervised by a competent physician who is also a physiologist. Stick to aspirin and cortisone, gold and anti-inflammation drugs. You may have no improvement, you may suffer side reactions from the drugs, but you will at least—as you take your medicine and learn to live with your arthritis—have the satisfaction of knowing that you patronized scientific medicine and avoided quackery.

An interesting point, which should let physicians know that Dr. Kaufman's therapy is valuable and owes nothing to the power of suggestion, is the improvement in the sedimentation rates of the patients he treats with niacinamide. This is a blood test which is widely used as an index of pathological conditions in the body. Normalization in that test is, of course, an indication that the body is moving away from pathology and toward well-being, which makes it fascinating that the sedimentation rate in Kaufman's patients runs a parallel course with the joint range index: as mobility is restored to the joints, the blood test moves toward the normal. A typical case showing this is that of a sixty-eight-year-old woman with extremely severe rheumatoid arthritis. Her initial response to the niacinamide therapy was pronounced, but subsequently slowed up. Although she was eating enough protein, her calorie intake was so low that an undue amount of the protein was being used as fuel, rather than being available for repair of tissues and joints. Dr. Kaufman increased her niacinamide intake to the top level of four grams (4,000 milligrams) daily. Her sedimentation rate fell sharply, mirroring reduction of the inflammation which is part of rheumatoid arthritis. But other indexes revealed other improvements. The patient's hemoglobin and red blood cell count rose, and simple arithmetic indicated that she had managed to manufacture twelve grams of additional hemoglobin in her blood solely as a result of the treatment with niacinamide. Actual measurement showed a dramatic decrease in the swelling at her knees.

Among Dr. Kaufman's voluminous data, there is a comparison of an untreated and aging population with a group treated with niacinamide. The joint range index for the untreated population gradually worsens, seeming to confirm that stiff joints and aging are linked. But in the niacinamide-treated group, with the same age distribution, improvement takes place in all age groups, with larger doses of niacinamide used, of course, in the treatment of more severe symptoms of impaired joint mobility.

Kaufman does not propose—and I do not picture—that niacinamide therapy is a panacea. There are a number of conditioning factors which determine how much benefit, if any, can be achieved with the vitamin treatment. As the physician puts it, niacinamide, in the proper doses at the proper intervals, can cause significant improvements in joint mobility in arthritics if:

1. They are eating diets adequate in protein and calories.
2. Their joints have not been excessively—irreversibly—damaged, by aspects of their work, life-style, or whatever.
3. Their joints have not been so damaged by the arthritis prior to treatment as to leave no chance for improvement.

Point 1, a diet adequate in protein and calories, has been previously explained, but because of ill-founded scare stories about high-protein diets, let me recapitulate the reasoning behind this provision. When the intake of calories is not adequate—which it isn't, in many people—the body will turn to other sources for its energy needs. Thus, while carbohydrate (starch, sugar) and fat are ordinarily the body fuels, protein begins to substitute when there isn't enough of the starches, sugars, and fats to meet energy needs. That protein is needed for repair of tissues, which includes joints, and the diversion of it to fuel may deprive the body of the necessary rebuilding substances which come from foods like meat, fish, fowl, cheese, eggs, milk, and dairy products other than butter and cream.

The case histories you have read cover periods of niacinamide treatment ranging from a few months to about three years. The skeptic at this point may be justified in asking if the treatment is continued, do the benefits hold? It is here that we see the dividends which accrue when a physician devotes many decades to a type of treatment, for Kaufman's records indicate what eventuates with as many as twenty years of uninterrupted niacinamide treatment.

Addressing the question whether niacinamide therapy can yield improved joint mobility for ten years or more, the doctor gives us examples of cases which represent as many as twenty years of uninterrupted treatment. He begins, though, with a woman who is a backslider, for she started and stopped treatment four times. Each time she went back to niacinamide, her joint range index improved, and it worsened each time she stopped, returning to what it would have been, perhaps, if she had never had the vitamin treatment.

Between the ages of fifty-two and seventy-two, a mother took niacinamide for moderate joint dysfunction. By the third year of treatment, her joint dysfunction had literally disappeared. For the next seventeen years of uninterrupted niacinamide treatment, the flexibility of her joints was that of a healthy fifteen-year-old girl, and stayed at that level beyond her seventy-second year.

Similarly, a thirty-two-year-old man began treatment with moderate joint dysfunction which improved for seventeen years of niacinamide therapy, to the point where in this long period, his joint range index remained between slight dysfunction and none at all.

Trauma to the joints has been mentioned as a limiting factor in response to the niacinamide treatment. It is illustrated in the history of a golf enthusiast, sixty one years of age, who used his hands in hard work, too. His joint range index was in the severe classification at the beginning of treatment, but improved to moderate despite the fact that he continued to insult his hands with his golf and his work. That improvement continued for more than sixteen years.

Some important points emerge as one studies the decades of Dr. Kaufman's research. It is obvious, even to the prejudiced, that the physician has demonstrated that there *is* a vitamin therapy that benefits hypertrophic and rheumatoid arthritis. It is clear that the therapy can be used for very long periods without side effects. Dr. Kaufman's conclusion seems to be reasonable: there is no basis for supposing, he writes, that such benefits could not be maintained for an entire life span. It is apparent that this type of orthomolecular (the right molecule) treatment can refute the ancient belief that joints must stiffen as one grows older, whether or not one is arthritic. The physician who studies Dr. Kaufman's findings will inevitably come to the conclusion that niacinamide also confers other benefits in retarding degenerative changes usually considered inevitable in the aging organism. For example, Kaufman was curious about the effects, if any, of the vitamin on the walls of vessels in the eye. In the process usually blamed on aging, the walls of the retinal vessels become less transparent with the years. This is often used as an index of the progression of atherosclerosis (pathological hardening of the arteries) in the brain and elsewhere. But in the niacinamide-treated arthritics, the physician recorded a slow but progressive tendency for transparency to return to the walls of these blood vessels. He also finds that the incidence of strokes was lower in such patients than the expected incidence in their age groups. All this adds up to a simple statement: what happens to the blood vessels in the eye, as age increases, is reversible—perhaps to a significant degree, with niacinamide therapy over a long period.

Throughout this book, I have made it more than clear that I professionally resent the misinformation dispensed by the arthritis orthodoxy on the subject of nutrition in the prevention and treatment of this group of diseases. Let me now direct your attention to the type of propaganda to which both the public and the professions are subjected, masquerading as the scientific truth. Thus Kaufman quotes an eminent and well-respected pharmacologist as saying that "vitamins are used by the medical profession and the laity under the mistaken impression that larger amounts than the minimal daily requirement will promote optimal health."

Comment: the minimum daily requirement for pigs and rhesus monkeys, set by the same authorities who dictate those for human beings, are up to *fifteen* times as high as those for people. Pigs and rhesus monkeys are expensive, and obviously, nothing should be spared in keeping them healthy.

The statement by the pharmacologist continues: "It is believed by critical authorities that most of the widespread use of vitamins by the population is wasteful and that the benefits claimed by many persons must be due to a placebo effect." "Placebo effect"—healing by the power of suggestion. Can you picture suggestion so overwhelming that it keeps arthritic joints functional and free of pain for twenty years?

Dr. Kaufman, in response, points out that he has demonstrated with objective measurements that niacinamide alone or combined with other vitamins can improve joint mobility, improve impaired muscle strength, increase maximum muscle working capacity, restore or improve the sense of balance, and ameliorate certain mental syndromes found in the over-fifty-five age group.

Demonstrating that the prime mover in his nutritional treatment was the niacinamide, the doctor tells us of eleven "stubborn" patients who refused to take the vitamin treatment, and insisted that the doctor put them on "the best possible diet." This he did, and in periods ranging up to a year of such treatment with good diet alone, none of these patients enjoyed an improvement in joint range index. There were other patients who reduced their doses of niacinamide or tried to substitute an ordinary multiple vitamin supplement, of the one-per-day variety. Whatever improvements they had achieved from the niacinamide therapy they gradually lost. Patients who refused to take anything, including niacinamide (after being on it for a significant period of time), suffered a worsening of their joint disabilities, which ultimately brought their joint range index down to the pre-niacinamide-treatment level.

Dr. Kaufman, with understandable emphasis, calls niacinamide "a most neglected vitamin." It is appropriate. He uses it to help arthritis, which, plied with ineffective drugs of dubious safety, is actually a most neglected disease.

7

A Nonrestrictive Arthritic Diet

What if you have arthritis, you don't have hypoglycemia, you're not allergic, you tolerate the nightshades, and all you need is a well-balanced diet?

There are three standards by which any national diet must be judged:

1. It must support efficient reproduction. If the diet doesn't allow people to be born—healthy— there's no point in examining it further.
2. It must support growth of the young in good health, and maintenance and repair of the mature, in good health.
3. It must maximize resistance to illness, facilitate recovery when people do become ill, and make for maximum longevity.

Since there are some fourteen nations in which babies have a better chance to arrive in good health and grow up, than they do in the United States, our national diet obviously fails to support efficient reproduction. It also fails to maintain good health and, contrary to what you've been told, it has *not* prolonged the life span for adults. What improvement there was came from the antibiotic victory over infectious diseases, but that doesn't make death from heart disease, hypertension, atherosclerosis, and cancer any more palatable.

All this explains why for a good diet for an arthritic with

no restrictions on choices of foods, I have selected a diet which I know supports efficient reproduction. I know, because it was tested on a thousand pregnant women, whose histories and babies were compared with those of a control group. So it is that you don't have to be female and pregnant to profit by the kind of good nutrition described in the following menu framework. Considerations of weight gain may lead you to minimize portions of carbohydrates, but don't do that with protein foods. Personal dislikes or favorites in foods may lead you to make some substitutions, but be sure that you substitute like for like. Fish can be eaten instead of meat, or cheese instead of fish, but you can't substitute bread or cereal for a protein food, or a starch for fat. Your daily intake would be as follows:

> One eight-ounce glass of unstrained fruit juice, preferably citrus.
>
> One serving of fresh fruit, unpeeled. Wash thoroughly.
>
> Two cups of cooked vegetables, slightly undercooked.
>
> One cup of mixed green salad, with a dressing containing vegetable oil of choice. Be sure it doesn't contain preservatives, such as BHT or BHA, or partially hydrogenated fats.
>
> Three squares of butter.
>
> One serving of oatmeal, whole-wheat, or other whole-grain cereal, with a teaspoonful of added wheat germ, and one tablespoon of bran.
>
> Two eggs.
>
> Six ounces of lean meat, fish, or fowl, with emphasis on liver—any type—kidney, sweetbreads, and other organ meats.
>
> Four slices of whole-wheat, whole-rye, or whole-corn bread or muffins. (This doesn't mean commercial rye bread or pumpernickel, "wheat

bread,'' or other types which are actually overprocessed.)

For dessert: whole gelatin, junket, custard, stewed fruit, plain yogurt with added fruit, fruit whip. No conventional pastries, no commercial ice cream.

Conventional spaghetti, macaroni, and noodles should be avoided. Buy high-protein types, which are made with added gluten and wheat germ.

Brewer's yeast, wheat germ, dried skimmed milk, and soy flour can be added to appropriate recipes, which range from meat loaf to baked foods.

Newcomers to nutrition should consult *The Carlton Fredericks New and Revised Cook Book for Good Nutrition* (New York: Grosset & Dunlap, 1974).

Supplements should at least include multiple-vitamin, multiple-mineral, and Vitamin B Complex concentrates. Other supplementary nutrients may be used, as listed in the text and in the Appendix.

WHEN THE BODY'S THERMOSTAT IS SET TOO LOW

Much of the attention to glandular disturbances in arthritis has been devoted to the pituitary and adrenal glands, since their antistress effects are critical in rheumatoid arthritis. The thyroid gland has not received enough attention, perhaps because its malfunction is rarely severe, and the symptoms are so common that they are (almost) regarded as being normal. If as an arthritic at the age of fifty-five or sixty you are constipated, catch too many colds, have dry skin, dry hair, and brittle nails, you yourself (as well as the incautious physician) may consider these slight disturbances as average (and therefore normal) penalties for growing old.

If you complain of feeling cold when other people don't of needing more blankets than your spouse, or of tiring more quickly than you should, these symptoms, too, may be assigned to the impaired circulation of the aging process. But every symptom I've listed in this paragraph can be caused or aggravated by an underactive thyroid gland. Moreover, the conventional tests for thyroid function—if needed such tests are ordered—may *not* indicate that the thyroid is misbehaving. Which calls for an explanation.

The conventional blood tests for thyroid function measure the amount of thyroid hormone precursor—the building material for the hormone—and the amount of the hormone in the blood. This is somewhat analogous to attempting to test the function of an automobile motor by measuring the amount of gasoline in the tank and the fuel line. Obviously, you'll have to turn the motor on. That is the basis for a simpler test, which costs nothing—and which is ignored in the United States, but used widely in Europe. It has been recommended here by Dr. Broda Barnes, an authority on thyroid function. Simply stated, the test requires that you shake down a fever thermometer before going to sleep. When you awaken, before you leave your bed, place the thermometer under your arm—in the armpit—and keep it there for ten minutes. Do this for three days in succession. If you are a menstruating woman, do it on the first day of the period. If the temperature averages below 97.8°F., and you have some of the symptoms listed above, the odds are long that your thyroid is underactive. If the temperature is above 98.2°F., it may indicate an overactive thyroid, but I should anticipate that this would be rare in arthritics. Conversely, if you are both arthritic and a hypoglycemic, I should expect your temperature reading to be low—particularly, if you're female. If the reference to "female" puzzles you, let me explain that in many hypoglycemic women, arthritic or not, there is a rise in estrogenic (female) hormone activity, and this hormone and the thyroid are antagonists. While it has nothing to do with arthritis, I can't resist, with my interest in prevention, telling you that an underactive thyroid is a risk factor of breast cancer; and high estrogenic hormone activity is also an invitation to it.

It is a commonly held misconception that iodine is the whole story of nutritional support for the thyroid gland. Not so: chronic deficiency in Vitamin B_1 can cause irreversible thyroid underactivity. Also, there are foods which, taken in excessively large amounts, are antithyroid. These include the cabbage family—Brussels sprouts, kale, rutabaga—liver, and soy products. Large doses of Vitamin A, PABA, or Vitamin E may have antithyroid effects. This does not mean that supplements of these factors are tabooed, but that very high doses must be avoided by those who have this thyroid problem.

Until the excessive intake of salt by Americans made it unwise, we used to recommend iodized salt as a source of that essential. With salt intake an average of five to seven times the requirement, and linked with potassium deficiency as causing hypertension in the susceptible, a multiple mineral supplement which supplies iodine is preferable. Kelp tablets can also be used. Doses of iodine need to be conservative, and medical guidance or at least the instructions on the labels of multiple mineral or kelp supplements should be strictly followed. If the thyroid gland refuses to respond to iodine and Vitamin B_1, the physician may resort to doses of thyroid hormone. Despite widespread use of synthetic thyroid hormone preparations, it is my impression that natural thyroid, such as marketed by Armour, is preferable. Dr. Broda Barnes strongly prefers this form, but your physician will of course make the decision. It is of interest that Barnes claims for thyroid treatment a marked rise in resistance to heart attacks. Whether or not that dividend results, it is obviously important to an arthritic that the thermostat of the body—the thyroid—function properly. Otherwise, the symptoms it causes merge with those associated with the arthritis, adding to your fatigue and feelings of ill-being.

The statistical chance that you are a victim of an under-active thyroid is far from being astronomically small. The medical literature indicates that *obvious* underactivity is present in some 3 percent of males and 10 percent of females, and those figures don't include a vast number of people with slight, and yet debilitating, thyroid underactivity. The authorities suggest that your intake of iodine should be about 100 micrograms daily—a tenth of a milligram. Against this are studies at the University of Alabama, on a group of doctors and their wives, which show that higher intake—above the 100-microgram level and going as high as more than 4,000 micrograms—is meaningfully correlated with improved health. This is another way of saying that the more healthy practitioners tended to be ingesting more iodine than the authorities recommend. The figures indicate that 1,000 micrograms, rather than 100, may be the ideal daily ration. Until you discuss this with your physician,* follow the label instructions, as I previously suggested, on iodine supplements.

ZINC

There is direct evidence that zinc deficiency is involved in rheumatoid arthritis. I have already cited studies in which the administration of the metal has yielded benefits to such patients. But zinc deficiency isn't confined to them. The American intake of zinc, in part due to the persistent removal of the nutrient from popular overprocessed foods, is unsatisfactory. We are so close to nationwide deficiency in

*If your physician is curious about the research leading to recommendation of higher iodine intake, he can communicate with Dr. W. M. Ringsdorf, Jr., or Dr. Emmanuel Cheraskin, at the University of Alabama Medical School, Birmingham, AL 35233. I am *not* recommending queries from nonprofessionals.

this important factor that we have no margin whatsoever for emergencies. Dr. Carl Pfeiffer has pointed out that the American Orthodox Jew who fasts on Yom Kippur, a high holy day, can be identified easily, simply by looking at his fingernails, where white spots will appear as the price of zinc deficiency aggravated by *one single day* of abstinence from food. Obviously, our national diet leaves us with no reserves of the metal on which we can draw when, for whatever reason, our daily supply is interrupted. Similarly, the marks blamed on stretching in pregnancy—which so often appear before there has been any stretching—have been attributed in part to zinc deficiency induced or aggravated by the demands of the unborn; and many pregnant women also show white spots on the nails. Another clue to zinc deficiency appears when we take one of the antibiotics which interferes with the utilization of the nutrient. Though we blame the loss or blunting of the senses of taste and smell which may follow an infection on the infection itself, an induced zinc deficiency may frequently be the actual cause, for the metal is indispensable to our ability to taste and smell.

Since there is evidence from animal experiments that zinc deficiency can directly cause enlargements or deformities of bone, parallel to those blamed on arthritis in human beings, trial of medication with zinc in arthritis was obviously logical, the more so because the metal is important to the connective tissue which is weakened in many arthritic conditions. Such trials have yielded benefits in rheumatoid arthritis. One would expect this, even if connective tissues were not involved, for zinc is an important factor in carbohydrate metabolism, and you have already read that many rheumatoid arthritics have disturbed tolerance for starches and sugars. Dividends from zinc administration in arthritics have included improvement in tender, stiff, and swollen joints, and in the ability to walk rapidly. Grip strength did not respond, but you will recall that it was one of the functions which Dr. William Kaufman restored with doses of niacinamide.

A Nonrestrictive Arthritic Diet

Of late, zinc supplements have been used to treat refractory acne. This effect on the skin derives from the action of zinc in increasing the amounts of three amino acids in skin. The same amino acids are vital to normal connective (collagen) tissue. Readers with long memories will recall that Vitamin A has been recommended in acne for some time, but may not know that an interrelationship has been found between that vitamin and zinc—so much so, that zinc treatment of disturbances of the senses of taste and smell has been made more effective by simultaneous use of Vitamin A. All this underscores the importance of using nutritional factors together, rather than searching for one magic vitamin, protein, fat, or mineral.

As the aging process may be blamed for symptoms actually caused by hypoglycemia, and arthritis may be indicted for symptoms deriving from allergy or an underactive thyroid, so may zinc deficiency go unrecognized, or its effects attributed to other causes. It is an article of faith that older people don't heal as quickly as the young. It is an article of biochemistry that zinc deficiency will interfere with healing.Even some of the disturbances of mental performance which are blamed on the calendar may possibly derive from zinc deficiency. The skeptical should read the story of Fran, a little girl given to unprovoked outbreaks of uncontrollable and violent rage, whose parents noticed that she quieted down dramatically after a meal of her favorite food: fried oysters. Knowing that oysters are our richest source of zinc, Dr. Pfeiffer then demonstrated that the same tranquilizing effects on Fran followed doses of a zinc supplement, and closed the case by showing that the maniacal outburst returned when, without her knowledge, Fran was given a placebo—a tablet identical in appearance with her zinc supplement but containing none of the metal.*

I have given you these data on conditions other than

*Dr. Carl C. Pfieffer, Brain Bio Center, Princeton, N. J.

arthritis which involve zinc metabolism to underscore not only the importance of this nutrient, but how essential it is for the arthritic to assure adequate intake. Remember that under the term "arthritis" hides a whole group of diseases of connective tissues—collagen—involving some 95 percent of all Americans over the age of sixty, and remember that this connective tissue leans heavily on zinc and Vitamin C for its integrity.

When you survey your dietary habits, as an average American, in terms of zinc sources it will look almost as if you had set out to avoid intake of this nutrient. It's concentrated in shellfish, not only oysters, and in whole grains— whole wheat, whole rye, whole corn, brown rice, whole buckwheat, and other grains which have not been overprocessed. It is generously provided by eggs and liver— which the low-cholesterol faddists have tried to remove from your diet. Question: looking at that list of foods, how often do you eat those which fortify your zinc intake?

Zinc supplements are, of course, available, and I have already indicated that it would be wise to supplement your intake. Leave therapeutic doses to your physician, but insure your diet by taking at least fifteen milligrams of zinc daily, or, if digestive efficiency and absorption are questionable, up to fifty milligrams daily. You must read labels carefully, for the weight of the tablet isn't identical with the amount of zinc it supplies. Thus a 100-milligram tablet of a zinc salt— say, zinc sulfate—doesn't supply 100 milligrams of zinc, for a good part of the molecule is the "sulfate." The label should tell you how much *elemental* zinc the tablet or capsule yields in the recommended dosage. Don't pay astronomical prices for "chelated zinc." It is better absorbed than nonchelated forms, like zinc sulfate, but ordinary zinc gluconate is less expensive and very well utilized. Remember that the supplementary dosages I have listed here are for dietary insurance. For therapeutic purposes, your medical nutritionist may increase the amount recommended.

VITAMIN D

There are nutritionists and physicians who believe that the public is being overdosed with Vitamin D in such fortified foods as milk, and strongly believe that the recommended intake of the vitamin should be reduced from 400 units daily. Against this, there are the accurate reports that the housebound elderly—which would certainly include many arthritics—who are deprived of sunshine and do not take supplementary Vitamin D consistently, suffer the effects of low levels of the vitamin in the body. There are also reports that arthritics have benefited from the use of cod-liver oil, certainly a time-honored supplementary source of Vitamin D, Vitamin A, and other important nutrients. (In writing this, I am distinctly not endorsing the claim, made by some nutritionists, that cod-liver oil "lubricates" the joints.) Some consideration, in evaluating these arguments, should be given to the forgotten use, decades ago, of very high doses of Vitamin D in the *treatment* of arthritis—doses running as high as 150,000 units daily and more. I believe that any benefits derived from this drastic treatment probably came from stimulation of glandular function by the vitamin, for Vitamin D is known to stimulate the pituitary gland. That is one reason for the effect of the vitamin in preventing hibernating animals from their long winter sleep. At any rate, I have long thought that we discarded some important nutritional benefits when we dropped the use of cod-liver oil, and began to concentrate only the Vitamins A and D from fish liver for supplementary use. For one thing, the oil has a remarkable effect in controlling blood cholesterol, an action of which infants are now deprived. I vote for a reasonable use of a high-grade cod-liver oil by arthritics—particularly the housebound and others who for one reason or another have limited exposure to sunshine. The Vitamin A in the oil has, if you remember the discussion of zinc in this text, a cooperative action with that metal in the body.

VITAMIN E

For years, orthodox medicine—personified by the American Medical Association—has downgraded Vitamin E, beginning by denying that it is essential to human beings, conceding essentiality but denying the possibility of deficiency in it, and emphasizing that no disorder has ever been traced to lack of the vitamin. The phrase of the AMA was that "Vitamin E is a vitamin in search of a disease." The public, impressed by the purported authoritativeness of this medical society (which actually has been defined as a labor union, by a federal court, and which does no research at all), was and is puzzled about the vitamin. Actually, the medical society spake with forked tongue, for while these negative remarks went to the mass media, in the journals of the AMA were many reports emphasizing the importance of Vitamin E in human nutrition. These included the use of the vitamin as a substitute for dangerous estrogen in the treatment of menopausal sweats and flushes, use of the vitamin in the prevention of a blinding eye disease in premature babies, an action of the vitamin in preventing a type of cataract, helpfulness of the vitamin in restoring circulation in arthritics, and, though not finally, the importance of Vitamin E as an antiaging and anticancer factor, the last discussed in glowing terms by a former editor of the *Journal of the American Medical Association*.

A full discussion of Vitamin E—in its own right, or as a factor helpful to arthritics—would require a separate book. No such book has ever been written, for those on the market tend to concentrate on the use of the vitamin in a specific therapeutic application, such as heart disease. Suffice it to say that the vitamin stimulates the pituitary gland, an action important to rheumatoids particularly; it stimulates circulation; it strengthens blood vessels; it offsets some of the side reactions of drugs, including hormones, frequently prescribed for arthritics; and it reduces the needs of the cells for

A Nonrestrictive Arthritic Diet

oxygen. Space limitations forbid discussing its helpful effects in preventing thrombosis (clots) and phlebitis and thrombophlebitis, clearly demonstrated by a research group at Tulane University. By the same token, I can't explore the helpfulness of the vitamin in benign hypertrophy of the prostate, a disorder certainly common in the same elderly males who are the victims also of arthritis. But I do wish you to understand the antioxidant effect of Vitamin E, because that will dictate the form of the vitamin which should be chosen.

Vitamin E, together with Vitamin C, selenium, and sulfur-containing amino acids such as are provided by eggs, joins with lecithin in protecting our cells from the effects of what chemists call "free radicals." Without getting too technical, let me explain that these are vigorously active chemicals, possibly formed as a result of our universal exposure to cosmic rays (and X rays), which cause premature aging and death of the cells in which they interrupt vital processes, or derange them. That action of Vitamin E isn't shared equally by all forms of the vitamin. The type which is purchased by the public is called "alpha tocopherol." Whether this is the natural vitamin, or the synthetic—which is less potent—alpha tocopherol has the greatest beneficial effect on the heart cells, the greatest effect on cellular chemistry, but the least effect on the "free radicals" and on reducing the oxygen needs of the cells. The forms of the vitamin most effective against free radicals and most efficient in reducing oxygen needs are the beta, gamma, and delta tocopherols. To put it another way, in terms of cellular chemistry, the declining order of potency of forms of Vitamin E would be alpha, beta, gamma, and then delta tocopherols. In terms of anti-free-radical and antioxidant effects, that list reverses, and the declining order would be delta, gamma, beta, and alpha tocopherols. If all this is confusing, let it add up to a simple suggestion: don't buy alpha tocopherol as a Vitamin E supplement. Buy *mixed* tocopherols, which give you all four

145

forms. The potency will be stated in terms of alpha tocopherol alone, but I hope that some day the industry will give us label statements on how much of the beta, gamma, and delta forms are also present. Only in this form—mixed tocopherols—will you have a supplement which offers the chance of maximum dividends from raising your Vitamin E intake.

It has been widely reported that Vitamin E tends to raise blood pressure. This has been used as part of the scare tactics by food-drug industry spokesmen masquerading as consumer protectors. This effect does appear in a small group of Vitamin E users, and must be regarded as an idiosyncrasy of the subjects rather than a characteristic of the vitamin. The group tends to be hypertensive—meaning that their tendency to high blood pressure was obvious before they used the vitamin—and they tend to be elderly. These characteristics don't prevent physicians from giving such patients Vitamin E when they need it for a significant reason. They simply require that initial doses be small, and rises in the doses gradual, with monitoring of the blood pressure—which would be requisite regularly in hypertensives anyway. To make everything even clearer: I am writing this book a few months before my seventieth birthday. Not only has my Vitamin E supplement, as part of my list of antioxidants, kept me physiologically twenty years younger than my calendar age, but my blood pressure is 124/70. Obviously, I'm not alone among Vitamin E users in avoiding hypertension.

Another action of Vitamin E—one with which even the scaremongers don't seem to be acquainted—is its antithyroid effect. By that, I don't mean that the vitamin helps to create the symptoms of an underactive thyroid. If it did, I'd stop taking and recommending Vitamin E supplements. What it does is keep the underarm temperature low—at the level which ordinarily indicates low thyroid activity. Other low-thyroid symptoms don't appear. I'm inclined to regard that as a plus, rather than a minus, not only because the action, again, is demonstrated on only a small group of Vitamin E users, but because low body temperature is linked with longer life in every species studied. In that context, I should remind you that my good friend Dr. Richard Passwater has demonstrated a startling drop in the incidence of heart attacks in users of Vitamin E supplements—and the effect is directly linked with the duration and the potency of the supplementing, meaning that higher doses and longer term of usage are directly associated with increasing resistance to heart attacks.

The legumes—beans, peas—the whole grains, and wheat germ are richer sources of the vitamin. Wheat-germ oil, which I use to fortify other oils lower in Vitamin E, is perhaps the most concentrated natural source, though not enough to be used therapeutically.

If you test any group of Americans for adequacy of Vitamin E intake, using what is called the diene test, you will find that a majority of them aren't properly supplied. In part, this is due to the insensate overprocessing of our grains, which should be rich sources of Vitamin E. White flour is the classic example: overprocessing removes some 90 percent of the vitamin, and the bleaching of the flour removes most of what little is left. Therefore, I begin Vitamin E supplements, admittedly at a low level, as early as possible —in infancy, literally. For the adult under forty and in good health, I use mixed tocopherols with a potency of 100 to 200 international units. I double this for the healthy who are over forty, and may increase it for those with physical disorders, like arthritis, at any age, and very particularly for those who are over fifty-five and have the disorder, for the utilization of fats and fatty factors, like Vitamin E, doesn't improve with disease and certainly goes down hill as one ages. Often I give lecithin with the vitamin, since it helps utilization and has its own antioxidant effects to fortify those of the vitamin.

There are, I should note, medical nutritionists who use doses far above the levels I've discussed. They consider that they are employing the vitamin in a drug use, rather than as a nutrient. And they get results. Many of the responses aren't recorded in papers in medical journals, probably because the practitioners in nutrition, using Vitamin E, encounter them so often. For example, the muscle cramps to which both arthritics and nonarthritics are sometimes prone have been relieved with calcium supplements, but they also respond to Vitamin E. A team of Los Angeles physicians did report on one group of 125 patients, of whom more than half had suffered from leg cramps for more than five years, and some for more than twenty. One hundred and three out of 125 are now free of the cramps, thanks to 300 international units of Vitamin E daily. I give you this as an example of the losses suffered by arthritics when the arthritis orthodoxy condemns nutritional therapy—without a trial.

VITAMIN B₆

Vitamin B_6 has shared with a few other vitamins the title of "the forgotten factor." That applies not only to its use in arthritis, but in many other disorders. It is invaluable in the treatment of autistic children. It is a miraculous treatment, together with zinc, for a common type of schizophrenia. It is useful, again with zinc—the absorption of which it helps—in shrinking the enlarged prostate gland with which many (particularly elderly) men suffer. It wipes out a type of nausea in pregnancy. It may be an important factor in blocking one cause of atherosclerosis (hardening of the arteries). For want of it in infant formulas, babies have developed convulsions which caused permanent brain damage and mental retardation. It is linked with another convulsive disorder—epilepsy. The fact that absorption of zinc is greatly increased by Vitamin B_6 automatically makes this vitamin important in arthritis and other collagen disorders where zinc deficiency is part of the problem.

The history of Vitamin B_6 in the treatment of arthritis curiously overlaps the research of Dr. William Kaufman with niacinamide in that disorder, for the benefits claimed for B_6 and potassium therapies include many of those cited for treatment with the other vitamin. Dr. John Ellis is the pioneer in Vitamin B_6 therapy, but a mistaken hypothesis almost blocked his understanding of the value of the vitamin in arthritis. The confusion started when the physician tried the Morrison diet for arthritics. This is a low-fat, low-cholesterol diet, aimed at reducing blood cholesterol in the hope of halting or reversing hardening of the arteries. When the arthritics responded to the diet with improved circulation, Dr. Ellis was convinced that Lester Morrison's menus were ideal for arthritic disorders. Other improvements fortified his conclusion, for he saw remarkable dimunition of dizziness, tingling of arms and legs, violent muscle spasms, leg cramps, and immobility of the joints, particularly, the fingers. One can't blame Dr. Ellis for deciding that high animal fat was the chief culprit in the American diet, and particularly bad for arthritics. That theory led him to the point where he tried to persuade Texas cattle breeders to market "baby beef," which would contain less fat, and to concentrate on raising animals which would yield leaner meat. There was one disturbing fact that challenged the theory, however: the Morrison diet was not only lower in fat and cholesterol; it was also a better balanced diet, supplying better nutrition, with more vitamin-mineral intake than the menus of the patients had previously yielded. From a technical point of view, Dr. Ellis had the problem every researcher dreads: there was more than one variable operating in the nutritional equation, which immediately flawed the research. To sort matters out, he consulted with a well-known medical nutritionist, who may have startled him when she said flatly that she didn't accept the indictments of animal fats as *the* mischief-makers in the American diet. Which meant that the low-fat, low-cholesterol Morrison menus may have helped, but not necessarily on the basis of the restriction of animal fat intake.

There came a clue, presented by a man who had tried a

diet recommended by an insurance advertiser on the radio, in which there was emphasis on the use of peanut oil and pecans. He told Dr. Ellis that his muscles had become stronger, pain in his knees had become rare instead of constant, and his fingers "more limber and flexible." He explained that prior to the new diet, he couldn't clasp his fingers against the palms of his hands because "my fingers were stiff or fat or something." Here was a layman's description of reduction of stiffness and tenderness of the joints, and less edema (swelling). All this simply raised new questions: was it the peanut oil, or the pecans, or both?

The focus sharpened when more information, presented by an intelligent woman patient, reached Dr. Ellis. Because of diabetes and pain in the chest, she had been put on the Morrison diet, modified with the addition of peanuts and pecans daily. Her previous diet had been high in animal fat, low in carbohydrate, and rich in protein. Her response to the nuts was explicit. The pain in her chest became infrequent. Her fingers had all hurt, but on the new diet, only one was painful. All the fingers were less stiff. And the tingling in her fingers and arms—a symptom of thousands of patients—was gone. So were her leg cramps, and so was the weakness of her grip, which was so bad previously, she told the doctor, that she dropped dishes. On a subsequent visit, she reported that she was better able to tolerate cold weather and that she could now make a fist without pain. It had previously hurt so much that she cried when she attempted it.

Investigation of the variables distributed among a number of patients took time, but narrowed the number of possibilities. There was one patient who had used peanut oil, if you remember. Another had been exposed to a considerable amount of sunshine, which made it possible that his improvement was from ultraviolet light, rather than the nuts. Still others had been exposed to other factors which might have had an effect on their arthritis. One by one, these variables were ruled out, and the pecans became the focus of attention. Most nuts being good sources of Vitamin B Complex factors, as well as polyunsaturated oil, it became necessary to test the vitamins. The first patient was given the B Complex vitamins by injection, and in two weeks of such treatment reported significant progress in a symptom the doctor had deliberately avoided emphasizing: tingling of the hands. But this simply raised another question: which of the many vitamins in the B Complex was active against the neuritis in the fingers, the tingling in the hands and arms, and the cramps in the legs? Using a short sentence to condense years of the Ellis research, I can tell you that ultimately he traced the benefits to a single vitamin: B_6, pyridoxin. Later, he realized that the action in the body is linked with that of potassium.

The nursing staff in the hospital in Dr. Ellis's area were aware of his research and of the battle it initiated with the establishments in medicine, biochemistry, nutrition, and arthritis. Because they knew the value of his vitamin therapy and perhaps because, like many nurses, they were weary of medical obstructionism, they prefaced one of Dr. Ellis's books with a remarkable series of statements on the effects they had seen in patients treated with pyridoxin. They listed reduction of swelling of hands and fingers, improvement of coordination and flexion of fingers, improvement of sensation in the fingers with reduction in pain in finger joints, reduction of swollen feet (this in some of the nurses themselves), and reduction of chest pain in cardiacs, who were able thereby to reduce their doses of nitroglycerin. The nurses themselves also commented on relief of their premenstrual edema (swelling) when they took Vitamin B_6 in advance of menstruation. Leg cramps, they noted, were *frequently* relieved by Vitamin B_6. They emphasized that they were recording (and signing) these observations because they believed that other persons "should make use of Vitamin B_6."

Dr. Ellis verified his findings in every possible way, aware of the resistance his reports would meet. He actually had drawings made of the hands of one patient, before and after the vitamin therapy, clearly showing the improvement in the swelling and the deformity of arthritis. He took motion pictures before and after treatment with pyridoxin. He successfully treated hundreds and, he says, perhaps thousands of patients with rheumatism, whose response to Vitamin B_6 therapy was "spectacular." (To refresh your memory, why not go back to chapter 6, where I reprinted the note from Lenox Hill Hospital, advising the public that no diet and no dietary factor will help arthritis?)

With motion pictures to document his statements in an objective way rare in medical annals, Dr. Ellis spelled out the benefits his patients received from oral doses of Vitamin B_6, taken daily (in many cases, for periods ranging from four to eight years):

> Reduction of swelling in hands and fingers
> Improved range of finger flexion
> Improved coordination of finger movement
> Prevention of transient paralysis of the arms at
>   night
> Halting of leg cramps and muscle spasms at night

There were also subjective reports of improvements which obviously could not be captured on motion-picture film. These came after only six weeks of Vitamin B_6 therapy by mouth, and included:

> Improvement of perception and sensation in fin-
>   gertips
> Elimination of numbness and tingling in hands
>   and fingers
> Reduction or elimination of shoulder pain
> Improvement of shoulder and arm function
> Reduction of tenderness and pain in finger joints

The pioneering Texas physician was quick to apply his

findings to the painful swelling in the hands and feet of pregnant women. His notes do not record it, but there is evidence that there is a defect in the utilization of the vitamin in the first few months of pregnancy. He nonetheless speculates on the easy possibility that lack of Vitamin B_6 may be characteristic of many pregnant women. It is known to be in women taking the contraceptive pills, and since they simply mimic pregnancy, the reasoning is sound.

Dr. Ellis points out, as Dr. Kaufman does, that the onset of arthritic and rheumatic troubles is very gradual, and thereby goes unnoticed until overt symptoms appear. Edema of the hands and fingers precedes pain and stiffness in the shoulders, though at times there may be a sudden start of symptoms that have been labeled the "shoulder-hand" syndrome. He also acknowledges that it's best to start treatment as early as possible—older people tend to have less response to pyridoxin. While repeatedly commenting on the quickness of the action in many patients taking from 50 to 100 milligrams of the vitamin for periods as short as one week, he emphasizes that the vitamin isn't a drug, and its full action will never appear if you simply add it as a supplement to a poor diet. This is a way of saying that other nutrients are important, too, which echoes some of the experience of Dr. Kaufman.

In reviewing the research of Ellis and Kaufman, it becomes obvious again that nutrients interact. Diet should be complete, and so should supplements. In the case of vitamin B Complex concentrates, the need for complete therapy is obvious. The B vitamins are called a "complex" because they appear together in foods, which means that deficiency in a single factor, unless one is trying to achieve it with the specialized diets used for that purpose in laboratories, would be most unlikely. And in turn, that means that Kaufman's niacinamide therapy and Ellis's pyridoxin treatment should obviously be combined, and used with the entire Vitamin B Complex. This would bring in choline and other B vitamins, some of which Dr. Kaufman found helpful, if you remember.

Since vitamins ordinarily prevent what they cure, these responses to Vitamin B_6 add to the indictment against our overprocessed foods. It is a literal crime that only three of the vitamins removed from flour are restored in enrichment, for B_6 is one of those *not* restored. It is technological insanity to degerminate our starches—corn, wheat, rye, etc.—for the good reason that the germ is usually the site of Vitamin B_6 concentration, and what isn't there is in the bran, which is also removed.

Only one group in the population, Dr. Ellis says, would have to be cautious in taking Vitamin B_6. These would be people who have—or have a tendency toward—stomach ulcers. The vitamin may increase the production or the secretion of the gastric juices, which would be useful to many of us but a threat to the ulcerprone.

One final note for women: I have already commented on the action of pyridoxin in helping women to avoid water retention in the premenstrual week. The vitamin does something else: it stimulates the production of progesterone, widely regarded as the "antidote" for estrogen. Since estrogen is suspect as causing a type of breast, uterine, and ovarian cancer, as well as endometriosis, anything that stimulates production of the antagonist—progesterone—should be valuable to women. As an incidental dividend, the process started by Vitamin B_6 may shorten the menstrual.

POTASSIUM

Potassium deficiency is a complex subject. Specialists in hypertension now believe that our over-indulgence in sodium (salt) isn't critical *if* the potassium intake is adequate. There are a number of disorders in which potassium metabolism is disturbed, and a number of drugs which cause the body to lose potassium. Yet supplements of potassium can't be used without very close medical supervision, for there are forms of it, supposed to be safe, which have caused ulceration of the colon. I am inclined to draw on natural sources of potassium, with which such troubles aren't encountered. These include oranges, bananas, figs, raisins, dates, and, of course, as you know from the history of Dr. Ellis's research, nuts. Nuts would generally be the best source of natural potassium. Bananas are starch until they fully ripen, when they are largely sugar; the less ripe banana may occasionally be used, therefore. There are chelated forms of potassium available, the doses of which—because of more effective utilization—can be smaller, and the physician can guide you to these, if they are needed.

SELENIUM

In discussing the antioxidant property of Vitamin E, I mentioned Vitamin C, sulfur-containing amino acids, and selenium as having that effect too. Selenium has many remarkable actions in the body, among them favorable effects on the utilization of fats, antiaging effects, and the property of protecting against both heart disease and cancer particularly breast cancer. Yet selenium, like so many other nutrients, is removed from our popular processed carbohydrates and is, unfortunately, richly supplied by the foods which the low cholesterol diet forbids—eggs and liver, for instance. Selenium has been specifically recommended for arthritis.

To give one statistic: virtually in every area and every nation studied, low intake of selenium is associated with higher incidence of serious diseases. The ethnic groups and the nations who have a satisfactory selenium intake average about 500 micrograms (half of a milligram) of the mineral in the daily diet. Americans drop to about half of that, in many

155

cases, and even lower—and in the areas where selenium intake in this country is low, cancer and other diseases are much more frequent. (The cattle in such areas are, by government suggestion, given selenium supplements. Not the people, although their food comes from the same selenium-deficient soil.) The acid rain which derives from our use of fossil fuels drops sulfur compounds on the soil; this makes selenium unavailable to the plants, even when the soil content would normally be adequate.

If you use brewer's yeast in any significant amount, you will have a small supplementary selenium intake. If you prefer, you can buy concentrated yeast tablets, in which the selenium content has been raised to 50 micrograms per tablet. 100 micrograms—two tablets—would be a sensible supplementary level. Much higher amounts, which can sometimes be toxic, are administered in therapy by medical nutritionists. Cancer is one of the diseases experimentally treated in this way. I regard a selenium supplement as a sane investment, and not only for the arthritic. I wrote this book to try to answer your questions about nutrition in arthritis. May I ask one in return? Can you tell me why the arthritis specialists lump all this documented information with quackery, and refuse to review it, test it, or employ it as at least adjunct therapy in their practices?

Appendix

THE USE OF SUPPLEMENTS

We begin with a negative note: many rheumatoid arthritics have excessive levels of blood copper, and some have excessive iron. No multiple mineral supplement containing these two factors should be used if you are a rheumatoid arthritic, until you have checked with your physician. If either copper or iron is a problem (or both are), it may be possible to lower the levels by a medical technique called chelation, which your physician can explain for you. It involves dripping into the vein, three times weekly, a solution of an agent which will convey copper and iron out of the body. Simultaneously, it will remove calcium from plaques on the artery walls, thereby constituting a treatment for hardening of the arteries. Vitamin C and an amino acid, histidine, taken by mouth, also have a chelating action on copper and iron, and under medical supervision can be used to lower levels, if elevated, of these metals. Needless to say, the arthritic's condition improves if elevated copper or iron levels are lowered in rheumatoid arthritis.

Vitamin B_{12}

This vitamin is customarily given in large doses by injection. A substitute for injections, which bypass the poor absorption of the vitamin from the digestive tract, is the use of suckable lozenges of Vitamin B_{12}, which are dissolved under the tongue, where the vitamin is absorbed directly into the blood via the rich blood supply in that area. Five hundred micrograms daily is the usual supplementary amount. The chemical name is cobalamin.

Vitamin C

I have already expressed my preference for the sustained-release, matrix type of Vitamin C, in 500-milligram potency, two of which are used daily—morning and night. Higher doses are employed by many physicians, in conditions ranging from slipped disk to ankylosing spondylitis and types of arthritis. The vitamin is needed, as is zinc, for the maintenance of normal collagen (connective) tissue, which in arthritis is the site of disturbances. I prefer ascorbic acid to other forms of the vitamin.

Vitamin B$_6$ (Pyridoxin)

Fifty to 100 milligrams daily is the usual range of dosage —the lesser amount as a supplement, higher amounts for therapeutic purposes. The vitamin is used in 500- and 1,000-milligram doses, together with a similar amount of ascorbic acid (Vitamin C) to help to control cerebral (addictive) allergies.

Bioflavonoids

These are available as citrus bioflavonoids, hesperidin, hesperidin chalcone, and rutin. My preference is for the citrus bioflavonoids, which are employed as supplements in doses ranging from 1,000 to 3,000 milligrans (one to three grams) daily.

Vitamin E (Mixed Tocopherols)

Supplementary doses range from 100 to 400 international units daily. Multiples of these doses may be employed by the physician for therapy.

The Use of Supplements

Pantothenic Acid

This vitamin appears in supplements in several forms, among them pantothenol and calcium pantothenate. Actions are identical for all forms. Supplementary amounts range from fifty to 100 milligrams daily, but medical nutritionists may employ up to a gram (1,000 milligrams) daily to build resistance to stress by stimulating the adrenal glands.

Zinc

In the form of zinc gluconate, fifteen to fifty milligrams of elemental zinc daily is employed as a supplement. High doses are sometimes employed medically.

Multiple Vitamins

These are the one-per-day type, although in supplements of natural origin, which tend to be less concentrated than the synthetics, one may have to take one or two tablets several times daily. Be wary of products with a very long list of ingredients; the label may look impressive, but frequently the quantities supplied of some of the nutrients are so small as to be without significance.

Niacinamide

All doses specified in accordance with the Kaufman protocol, based on the degree of joint damage, are therapeutic, and should be medically supervised. They may range from a few hundred milligrams daily, taken in divided doses, to 4,000 milligrams daily, also in divided doses.

Appendix

Digestive Enzymes

Instructions will be found on the labels of pancreatic enzymes, bromelin, and papain products for adequate supplementary dosage. Primarily these are intended to help the utilization of protein, although fat and carbohydrate will also be affected by the pancreatic substance.

Calcium

Supplements of this nutrient are frequently used to help reduce cramping of the legs. My preference is for calcium orotate, which is a highly utilizable form of calcium, thereby reducing the quantity which must be taken. As little as 150 milligrams of calcium from the orotate form may be enough, while from other sources, as much as 1,000 milligrams may be necessary. Since the "orotate" part of the compound is a large molecule, it may require a 500-milligram tablet of calcium orotate to yield 50 milligrams of calcium. You must read labels carefully.

Magnesium

This nutrient is also involved in muscular spasm, and very important in protecting the heart against stress. Magnesium orotate is probably the most efficient form to use as a supplement, in amounts yielding 200 to 300 milligrams of magnesium daily, in divided doses.

Desiccated Liver

Liver is available in capsules and tablets, as a supplement. It is valuable because it is a source of protein and Vitamin B Complex, thereby a useful supplement where liver function

162

is inadequate, as in hypoglycemia. There is no dose; this is food. A handful of tablets would be the prescription. Buy desiccated liver only if described as originating in Argentina, where cattle are not subject to the sprays and medications which concentrate in dried liver preparations. Liver allergy is frequent.

Brewer's yeast

This is to be distinguished from an inferior type, called torula yeast; and if the label isn't explicit, don't buy it. Brewer's yeast contains factors missing from torula yeast, including a selenium compound important to good health and to recovery from types of arthritis. Be careful if you have never used yeast, for it contains many substances which can be sensitizing for those who are allergic. Flatulence will ordinarily be your first warning of allergy to it. This, too, is food, which you will appreciate when I tell you that in severe malnourishment, medical nutritionists may order one quarter pound of brewer's yeast daily, coupled with the same amount of desiccated liver.

Selenium

Those who wish to know definitely their intake of this nutrient can use yeast which has been concentrated, in tablets, for selenium value. Supplementary doses of selenium range from fifty to 100 micrograms daily.

Glucose Tolerance Factor

The situation with this factor is the same as with selenium. It is a natural constituent of brewer's yeast. If, because of its favorable effects on carbohydrate metabolism, important thereby to diabetics and hypoglycemics, you want to know that you're taking a definite amount of the glucose tolerance factor, you will find that, like selenium, it is available in concentrated yeast form, in tablets yielding about fifteen micrograms of the factor. The recommended supplementary amount is thirty micrograms daily for people under forty and double that for those who are older. Carbohydrate tolerances don't improve as you age, they deteriorate; hence the larger dose for the people over forty. The glucose tolerance factor combines chromium in a complex way with other nutrients. Don't buy chromium salts of any kind. Manufacture of the glucose tolerance factor within the body, starting with chromium, is uncertain.

PABA

This nutrient is part of the Vitamin B Complex and part of the molecule of folic acid. It is also the most active principle of GH3, the so-called rejuvenating formula from Rumania, but priced much more reasonably. It is available as para-amino-benzoic acid (PABA, in chemical shorthand) in fifty- and 100-milligram potencies, in the health food stores. The supplementary amounts would be in that range. PABA is also sold as a prescription drug, for the treatment of the pains associated with arthritic conditions, in which it is sometimes strikingly helpful—particularly in myositis and fibrositis. The prescription form is the potassium salt of PABA, which has the advantage of being more soluble, so that it dissolves and is utilized more easily in the digestive tract. The lowest potency available in this form is 500 milligrams, sold under the trade name of POTABA. Remember that a prescription is needed to purchase this, and that the dose should be set by your medical nutritionist. Side dividends from PABA may include pituitary stimulation, consequent stimulation of fertility, recoloring of gray hair, and longer retention of the characteristics of youth.

Choline

This nutrient has been mentioned in the text for two very different applications. Because choline is the precursor which the body uses to manufacture acetylcholine, which is needed for proper muscle function and tone, this nutrient is used as an adjunct to other vitamin therapies, such as niacinamide and pyridoxin, for arthritics whose muscle tone is poor. The biochemical pathways by which it is utilized require that choline, to improve muscle tone, be used with pantothenic acid and manganese. We have already discussed pantothenic acid, but face a problem with manganese, since there is a disturbance in the utilization of this mineral in some rheumatoid arthritics. Yet manganese is needed to support the immune system, via the thymus gland, and that system, as you now know, is misbehaving in rheumatoids. The decision in using manganese supplements must be made by the medical nutritionist, for some rheumatoid arthritics have such a slow turnover of the mineral that their blood levels are excessively high. However, choline alone, as Kaufman has reported, has been a stimulant to muscle tone, and not only in arthritics. The range of supplementary intake is from 500 to 1,000 milligrams daily, but more may be medically prescribed.

Choline has also been mentioned in this text as part of the formula used with reducing diets, particularly the low-carbohydrate type, to help to redistribute fat, moving it from the problem areas which ordinarily don't respond to weight loss. (In this action, inositol and polyunsaturated fat are also helpful.) One thousand milligrams of choline are used daily for fat redistribution, but this must be accompanied by Vitamin E (mixed tocopherols), supplementary amounts of which have already been described, and by inositol. Inositol, which not only influences fat metabolism but normalizes the transmission of nerve impulses, is used in 500-milligram daily supplemental amounts, though more may be used by medical nutritionists. Inositol, Vitamin E, and choline are also used to reduce estrogen activity in women subject to cystic breast disease and to uterine fibroid tumors.

In some individuals, intestinal bacteria attack choline, breaking it down and making it useless to the body. Such individuals will detect a fishy odor when given choline supplements. The problem is overcome by shifting to the use of lecithin, a natural factor involved in fat metabolism, which contains as part of its chemical structure both choline and inositol. In the past, lecithin was too low in choline to be useful, the required dose for this purpose being too high. However, as a result of the discovery that high-choline lecithin is useful in treating senile changes in the brain, the industry has now produced a high-choline lecithin, at least three times as rich in choline as the former product. One must look for "triple strength" lecithin capsules, or for a label indicating a 35 percent content of phosphatidyl choline.

Vitamin A

Much nonsense has been written about the toxicity of Vitamin A, a point adequately explored in this book. Anything is toxic if doses are too high. Up to 25,000 units of Vitamin A daily has never been accused of toxicity. Indeed, University of Alabama nutrition researchers report that the actual requirement for the vitamin in some people is as high as 33,000 units daily. The allergic may have a problem with Vitamin A derived from fish-liver oil, if sensitive to fish, which would also preclude the use of cod-liver oil. Such problems can be solved by shifting to Vitamin A from plant sources—a typical example being 10,000-unit capsules of beta carotene, which are commercially available, largely from mail-order vitamin suppliers. Let me reiterate my preference for cod-liver oil for arthritics, if tolerated, in the dosage recommended on the label. These oils aren't uniform in Vitamin A content, and a high-grade oil, rich in the vitamin, should be chosen.

You may have heard the term "supernutrition." The use of the supplements, as outlined in this Appendix, will promote supernutrition *if* the basic diet is as good as it can be made. Remember that there are unidentified nutrients in food which can't be supplied in supplements, a good example being the anti-fatigue factor in liver. We know it's there, but can't find it and identify its structure. Yet, given to well-fed animals, liver literally quadruples resistance to the fatigue of exhausting compulsory exercise. All this explains my earlier admonition: don't use the supplements to license a bad diet. Whatever benefits you gain—and you *will* gain some—will be far less than you could have achieved if you had mended your food habits.

HYPOGLYCEMIA DIETING

As in recent years consumer advocates have multiplied like the green bay tree, so have authorities in nutrition, dispensing "the ideal diet" to regain good health and the equally ideal diet to maintain it. Hypoglycemia has perhaps invited more of their attention and more of their dogmas and generalizations than most other topics in nutrition. I have listened to vegetarians who not only insist that a low-protein vegetarian diet is *the* sovereign remedy for low blood sugar, but assure the public that high protein diets actually poison human beings. (They are too new to the field of nutrition, apparently, to recall that Vilhjalmur Stefansson enjoyed improved health under medical supervision with a diet comprising only meat and fat.) I have winced as high-carbohydrate enthusiasts urge low-fat, low-protein diets, crammed with unprocessed starches, on everyone—including hypoglycemics. Let me state my position before I make suggestions for diets (note the plural!) in hypoglycemia. Emphasis on a single system of maintenance or therapeutic diet for all humanity is the mark of the obsessed, the incompetent, the profit-motivated, the misguided, or those who believe that their personal experiences with food represent the Eleventh Commandment. The generalizations I have just written apply to all those who generalize about nutrition, which means that they apply to hypoglycemia and, indeed, to all disorders responsive to nutritional therapies.

I gave my first lecture on hypoglycemia in 1944. It was dreadfully incomplete, but hindsight is so clear! Some of those now engaged in the attempt to stuff hypoglycemics with unprocessed carbohydrates and low-fat, low-protein menus were in 1944 unborn, clad in diapers, or trembling on the threshold of learning how to pronounce "hypoglycemia." In the more than thirty years which followed that first faltering lecture, I participated, as a consultant, in the diagnosis and treatment of thousands of hypoglycemics, and communicated constantly with medical nutritionists who were testing and treating tens of thousands more. You will forgive me if I am impatient with the all-knowing, as I am not with the ignorant. Ignorance is a challenge to an educator; opinionated ignorance is a disaster.

Those who are ignorant and manage to be opinionated present their diets as a cure for hypoglycemia. There is no cure; there *is* control. Once a hypoglycemic, you are potentially always a victim. Even here, individual differences operate, for there are those who can relax some of the dietary rules without penalty and those for whom hypoglycemia is like a type of alcoholism, where one single drink is the prelude to disaster. In presenting diet alone as cure or control for hypoglycemia, there are important omissions, for the condition doesn't arise from poor nutrition alone. The causes include heredity, stress, boredom, allergy, excessive intake of sugar and caffeine, malnourishment, and/or elevated insulin blood levels.

Another error—one I find repeated in many books and papers on the subject—blames hypoglycemia on a malfunction of the pancreas. Certainly, in the common type of low blood sugar, excessive production of insulin by the pancreas is a prime cause, but the liver is *always* involved, and actually is more vital to control of blood sugar than the pancreas.

Less frequent causes of hypoglycemia include sensitivity to certain amino acids, allergy to tobacco, cancer of the pancreas, failure of the adrenals, lack of the enzyme needed to split sucrose, inadequate production of a pancreatic hormone which raises blood sugar (glucagon), and failures of absorption from the intestinal tract. With these we are not here concerned—they are the problems with which the medical nutritionist must cope, via accurate diagnosis and appropriate treatment. We are targeted here on hyperinsulinism—excessive production of insulin—and liver dysfunction, which combine to lower blood sugar below the levels needed for proper function of the brain, the nervous system, and the body.

Heredity and stress should be considered together. Your genes may dictate a tendency toward diabetes, which may first be evidenced in hypoglycemia, followed by the second disease, or even by a combination of the two. It is possible to have diabetes and hypoglycemia, and it is possible successfully to treat even so potent a combination of disorders. Heredity also may determine your reactions to stress—indeed, the genes may determine that what is stress to one individual, to the point of being unbearable, may be tolerable or even enjoyable to another. There are other forces which operate there: at the end of your office day, you may find an hour in your darkroom, developing pictures, a grateful relaxation. A photographer would resent it, and find it stressful. Our principal problem with resistance to stress derives from the fact that the machinery in the body is gaited for short emergencies—for the attack of a saber-toothed tiger. It still operates that way, although most of the pressures of today are endless, or seem so. The body simply isn't equipped to handle crises of long duration—indeed, the term is inherently self-contradictory. Since the saber-toothed tiger reaction involves, among other responses, a whipping up of sugar reserves in the body, long-term emergencies create chaos in the body's sugar-controlling mechanisms. Thus you find both heredity and stress among the causes of hypoglycemia. The disorder emerges when the wisdom of the body can't cope with the demands upon it—can't successfully meet the challenge of a saber-toothed tiger who is your boss, wife, husband, or job, and never gives you a truce.

There is a corollary to what I have just written. If the sugar-regulating mechanisms of the body can't cope with the demands of constant stress, how well do you think they perform with the opposite situation: boredom, monotony, tedium, lack of a sense of challenge, lack of a sense of accomplishment? Answer: this is the emotional background for another type of low blood sugar. I mention it because diet alone will not control it. It is called "the flat curve"; it originates with a flat existence, and it must be treated psychiatrically as well as dietetically, or the brief improvement that accompanies better nutrition will promptly disappear.

Low blood sugar can be caused by allergy; allergy can be caused by low blood sugar. That interaction explains why some hypoglycemics derive no benefit from the diets they try. However well balanced, however well suited to control low blood sugar, no diet can be truly helpful if it contains foods to which the individual is sensitive. This, incidentally, explains why a high protein diet for hypoglycemia may fail, or produce limited benefit. Protein foods are often the trigger for allergic reactions—but so are the whole grains which are eulogized for hypoglycemics by vegetarians and high-carbohydrate fanatics. This underscores the importance of pursuing the tests for allergy which I've outlined, very particularly for the arthritic, whose symptoms will be worsened by both conditions: allergy and low blood sugar. This doesn't negate the fact that there are some individuals who profit by less protein than others need; and some who need more liberal carbohydrate intake than others can tolerate.

The restriction on sugar intake is mandatory for *all* hypoglycemics of the type we're describing. Sugars are ordinarily absorbed and metabolized very rapidly, which is an action opposite to what we want. We don't want the explosiveness of gasoline as a fuel, but something slower burning. This prohibition applies to all types of sugar—sucrose, glucose, fructose, honey, molasses, corn syrup solids, and so on. The topic of fructose needs exploration, primarily because of misconceptions fostered by the honey and the health food industries. Fructose has recently been presented as an ideal sugar for hypoglycemics and diabetics, and thereby for the entire public, on the grounds that it is metabolized more slowly than ordinary sugar (sucrose) and therefore doesn't stimulate excessive insulin production. This is true, but it sweeps indifferently by some unpleasant facts:

1. Fructose, like sucrose, is an overrefined, overprocessed "empty" food.
2. Like all sugars and starches, it requires metabolic help from vitamins and minerals—which it doesn't supply. It is in that sense a "parasite" like sucrose, raising vitamin-mineral needs while displacing foods which meet those needs.
3. There are hypoglycemics who have adverse reactions to fructose, and there are diabetics whose response to fructose is "spilling" sugar via the urine—a phenomenon physicians try to avoid.

On the plus side, if fructose is used in carefully minimized amounts, in a structured diet—which all adds up to medical supervision of the entire procedure—it helps to cope with the hypoglycemic's desire for sweets. There is still one reservation: it seems to lose its sweetening effect if used in hot foods and beverages. Dr. David Hawkins, of the North Nassau Mental Health and Nutrition Center, on Long Island, N.Y., informs me that when he is able to control the diet and limit the amount of fructose to two ounces daily, while eliminating other types of sugar as completely as possible, the procedure proves satisfactory in controlling hypoglycemia—particularly in children, who are likely to rebel when entirely deprived of their familiar sweets. For the adult —and the arthritic, for whom these notes are written—I am inclined to be cautious about the use of fructose, unless both the diet and the amount of the fruit sugar used are in accordance with Dr. Hawkins's recommendations.

Excessive intake of caffeine carries a double threat, both of them largely unappreciated by the public. Caffeine stimulates the adrenal glands, which explains part of the lift you experience from coffee, tea, chocolate, cocoa, and cola drinks. The hormones released by the adrenals, in response to the prodding by caffeine, include several which stimulate the liver into discharging stored sugar into the blood. When that happens, it is identical in its effects with those of swallowing sugar: the pancreas must deal with the rise in blood sugar, and the source of it doesn't matter. Thus the net result of drinking unsweetened coffee, oddly, is the same as taking sugar with it. If the pancreatic response includes release of too much insulin, the mischief follows. Caffeine in excessive quantities presents two other risks, one of which is caffeine poisoning, on the brink of which many coffee-swigging Americans totter. The symptoms include many of those of low blood sugar. Another side effect of caffeine involves women, for whom it may be a cause of breast cysts and, perhaps, of other disorders of the reproductive system. All this explains why the caffeine-containing beverages and chocolate are taboo for hypoglycemics—the more so if, as they usually are, they are accompanied by sugar.

The logical question every layman asks at this point is: what about saccharin? Forgetting about the thesis that it is a weak cocarcinogen, which it may be, the mischief of saccharin lies in the fact that its sweet taste in the mouth produces a genuine Pavlovian conditioned reflex in some hypoglycemics. That is to say, they react to the taste as if they had actually eaten sugar, and respond with production of insulin—which, of course, we are trying to minimize.

A word of cheer would seem to be important for those of you conditioned to large intake of sweets and unable to throw off the illusion that sugar is needed by man. When your nutrition is properly balanced for your needs, the appetite for sugar will decline.

There is a tendency for those who are weaning themselves away from coffee, tea, cocoa, and other caffeine sources to use herb teas. Mint and rosehip teas are, if not allergenic for you, satisfactory, but you must be careful with other types. Ginseng tea, for example, in reasonable amounts has not caused troubles, but in large quantities has produced adverse reactions. The doctrine to remember is: little dose, little trouble—unless you're allergic to the test beverage or food.

The diets which follow represent very low-sugar, low-carbohydrate, high-protein, relatively high-fat menus. "Relatively high fat" means what it says. The cereal, bread, and bakery establishments, via their captive professors in large universities, have spread the fear that low-carbohydrate menus always drive people into eating high fat, and high fat always creates hardening of the arteries or heart disease, or both. Careful studies show that the satiety value of high-protein, high-fat menus is so great that you automatically *don't* overeat. As for hardening of the arteries and heart attacks, the subject is too complex for analysis here. Suffice it to say that those authorities who formerly terrified the public by suggesting that a menu with butter, cream, and eggs should be recommended only by your friendly neighborhood mortician, are now telling us that only those who have a medically recognized problem in the body's management of fats need to restrict their intake of good foods on the grounds that they contain fat or cholesterol.

In using the following menus, keep in mind that they represent a starting point. In repeatedly emphasizing individual differences, I have really underlined the need to adjust menus to your needs, as experience dictates. Some of you will tolerate vegetable fat better than animal fat, though that can be overdone. Some will do better with homogenized fats —homogenized milk, whipped butter—than ordinary types. Some will thrive on the approximately sixty grams of carbohydrate (starch and sugar) in my menus. Some will need to raise that; some may need to lower it. In the ultimate analysis, no laboratory test tells us quite as much as the simple responses of the patient to questions like these (addressed to the arthritic who has hypoglycemia):

> Do you rise from sleep more refreshed?
> Is your appetite good?
> Has your resistance to fatigue improved?
> How's your skin, hair, nails?
> What's happening with stiffness, pain, or swelling of your joints?
> How's your elimination? (It should be effortless.)
> How's your sense of balance?

There are other queries, of course, but the sample gives you an idea of the value of subjective responses to a new type of diet.

The diet which follows is one which has been used by hundreds of physicians for thousands of hypoglycemics. Because of the low carbohydrate content—about sixty grams, which is perhaps 20 percent of the intake usual in many modern diets—some hypoglycemics will experience a mild *ketosis*. This is a reaction of the body whenever fat is the dominant energy source, and carbohydrate restricted. In a diabetic, the reaction would be very undesirable. In most reducing diets, whatever their composition, ketosis is encountered, for weight loss is accomplished by burning body fat, and thereby fat is being used as the prime energy source while carbohydrate intake is, as in virtually all reducing diets of whatever type, restricted. When the ketosis is mild, which it usually is, there is a slight feeling of malaise and fatigue, which is transient. Some people, however, are as individual in their reactions to ketosis as hypoglycemics are in reaction to sugar. In them, the ketosis may be more pronounced, and with that, the symptoms also. These are the persons for whom sixty grams of carbohydrate may be too little. For such hypoglycemics (and reducers), the physician will raise the carbohydrate level gradually until equilibrium is established, evidenced by disappearance of the symptoms of ketosis. That rise in carbohydrate intake must *never* be effected with sugars, fruit, honey, and the like, but always with complex carbohydrates (starches).

A short case history will tell you what happens if this advice isn't followed. A Los Angeles nutritionist, one of my students, overcame mental retardation and poor health when, as a youngster, he learned from my books that he might be a hypoglycemic—which proved to be so. He went on a sixty-gram-carbohydrate, high-protein, medium-fat diet (of the type which follows this discussion). On this, he achieved physical and mental health. Some years later, however, he complained to his physician and to me that he too often felt weak and had headaches. We immediately recognized the possibility of ketosis—of his carbohydrate intake being too low to meet his individual need. With the addition of two extra slices of whole-wheat bread and one medium-sized baked potato daily, he banished his symptoms.

The Basic Diet for Hypoglycemia

1. Choosing from the permitted foods, eat as much as you wish at and between meals. Your scale will tell you when portions, rather than frequency of eating, must be reduced.

2. If you are overweight and hypoglycemic, it is easily possible to lose weight while still controlling low blood sugar. The underweight will have more difficulty in simultaneously coping with both conditions, but many who

could not gain while suffering from hypoglycemia promptly did so when the disorder was brought under control.

3. Constipation, a common but gratuitous added problem for both arthritics and hypoglycemics, requires attention. Following the outline of the diet, you will find detailed instructions both for slow stool transit time and for constipation. It is important that these problems be solved, not only for the hypoglycemic and the arthritic in terms of their present difficulties, but for prevention of the diseases which originate with disturbed elimination. And laxatives are *not* the answer.

4. Choose your menus from the following:

Lean meat, fish, poultry, which can be broiled, baked, or roasted. Boiling is less satisfactory for retention of nutrients, and tends to reduce the efficiency of protein in supporting well-being. Avoid fried foods—particularly in restaurants, many of which employ filters to permit undesirable reuse of the same fat over and over again. Eat fish at least five times weekly. Use other protein sources, such as pressed cottage cheese, which is sold as farmer cheese and pot cheese.

Vegetables: spinach, chard, broccoli, kale, cabbage, cauliflower, string beans, squash, eggplant, asparagus, lettuce, tomato, cucumber. Please note that the nightshades in that list must not be used by those on the no-nightshade diet. To refresh your memory, the nightshades include peppers, white potato, tomato, and eggplant.

Fruit: apples, pears, peaches, melons, berries—fresh or water-packed canned. Those canned in their own juice represent fructose as a substitute for sucrose. Consult the discussion of fructose for guidance, but in any case, these carbohydrate-rich foods (and particularly fruits as a source of sugar) must be used with discretion until the hypoglycemia is under control, and cautiously increased thereafter. Eat oranges and grapefruit in moderation, and avoid candied dried fruit.

Beverages: do not use distilled water. If your local water supply is for any reason suspect, use a good bottled mineral water. Probably the best American water is that from Hot Springs, Arkansas. Use weak tea, the percolator types of de-caffeinated coffee, skim milk, unsweetened fruit juice. If you're the thirsty type, dilute your fruit juice with added mineral water. If you're starting with a concentrated juice, like the frozen types, add twice as much (mineral) water as the label instructions indicate.

Do not eat starchy foods, except for the allowed whole-grain bread. Do not use sugar and foods made with sugar—such as ketchup, doughnuts, Danish pastry, cookies, cake, pie, candy, chewing gum, sauces and gravies with added flour, and canned foods packed in either heavy or light syrup. Do not drink alcoholic beverages, regular coffee, strong tea, chocolate, cocoa, cola beverages, soft drinks made with sugar, other drinks made with sugar, corn syrup, corn-syrup solids, corn sweetener, and glucose. In the early stages of controlling hypoglycemia, also avoid saccharin. The conditioned-reflex action, mentioned earlier, is one reason, but there are, as you know, grave questions about the safety of using large quantities of this artificial sweetener. This doesn't prohibit the use of two or three saccharin tablets dai-ly, if you must.

Weigh yourself at the same time each morning. Consult your physician to decide your ideal weight, if you need that estimation. Reach it and stay there. The high-sugar diet which predisposes us to hypoglycemia, which in turn sharpens our desire for sweets, is often in the background of obesity.

Outline for the Day's Menus and Snacks

Note: from the preceding discussions, you should be aware that frequency of eating is as important as what you are eating. We are filling a hypoglycemic's depleted nutri-tion reserves, and we are trying to smooth the glucose-level curves, so that they don't dip deeply—as they may after hours without food—or refuse to go high enough to keep the brain, nervous system, and body adequately fueled.

Before breakfast: use your blender to make your high-energy drink—which is a must every day. Blend one tea-spoonful each of dry skim milk powder, protein powder, and brewer's yeast powder. Be sure the protein powder is a high-quality protein—ask your health food store owner; it should not be based on soy. Be sure the yeast is brewer's yeast and not torula yeast, which is undesirable. Liquify in water, unsweetened fruit juice, or fluid skim milk. The milk is least costly if reconstituted from skim milk powder. Add any flavoring, such as real vanilla, which pleases you. Vanilla, incidentally, will give you a sweet-type taste without the use of sugar.

Breakfast: fruit, approved list. Two slices of ham, or one slice ham and one egg (if your physician hasn't tabooed eggs). A substitute for ham is hoop cheese, which is pot cheese in the form used by bakers for making cheese cake. Farmer cheese in foil packages should not be used. One slice of whole-wheat bread or toast, with a small amount of butter. Water, weak tea, percolated decaffeinated coffee, with skim milk if desired. No sugar.

Two hours later: farmer, pot, imported Swiss or cheddar cheese. Water, weak tea, or skim milk. (All cheese imported from Switzerland is made from unpasteurized milk, which gives you the advantage of protein which has not been de-natured by heat. Expensive as imported cheese from Switzerland may be, it is usually much less costly than the native brands of cheese made from raw milk.)

Lunch: fair-sized portion of lean meat, fish, poultry, lean hamburger, or half cup of drained canned salmon, sardines, or tunafish. If you are concerned with lead intake from the solder used in canned foods, look for the two-piece cans, which are mechanically crimped, without solder. Repeat beverage from choices previously listed.

Two hours after lunch: repeat midmorning snack.

Evening meal: fruit or juice, as listed. Lean meat, fish, poultry, etc., as at lunch, with vegetables from approved list. No substitutions. Allowed beverage.

Before retiring: fruit from approved list, and piece of cheese.

For the overweight: the preceding recommendations are for the normal in weight. The entire diet can be converted into a reducing diet by adding a portion of mixed green salad with five teaspoonfuls of vegetable oil. Note that the oil isn't optional—it's mandatory. Without it, you won't lose weight; with it, most people do. Be sure the oil you select—corn, safflower, peanut, sesame—has no preservatives. Most of the supermarket oils contain BHT and BHA, which should be avoided. Buy your oil in the health food store.

For the constipated: there are those who have a problem with elimination which doesn't seem to involve actual constipation. It is called "slow transit time," which means that food residues may leave the body regularly, in bowel movements, but take too long to travel. In the course of that excessively slow journey, the residues are subjected to attack by bacteria in the bowel, which may convert some of the chemicals normal to the stool into alien substances which are very potent causes of cancer. We believe this to be the dominant reason for the terrible toll of bowel cancer in this country, for other cultures are free of the problem; and in those areas, stool transit time is much shorter than ours. The difference is dictated by the diet; more particularly, by a higher fiber intake. We lose fiber because our bread, cakes, cookies, cereals, and sugar are overprocessed, and the fibrous portion removed, to be fed to cattle and horses (which are expensive, and need health protection). The fiber which should be in our sugar is made into wallboard, or burned to fire the kettles in the sugar industry. As a result of a rather small deficit of fiber, we are also subject to appendicitis, constipation, hemorrhoids, diverticulosis, diverticulitis, and bowel cancer. Constipation is therefore a small red flag of warning, but when it's absent, you may still be the target for slow stool transit time and the opportunities it gives the bowel bacteria to make mischief.

If constipated, you can use the BAMBY plan which I proposed in a long-ago book on the high-fiber diet, which has helped hundreds of thousands of readers to solve the problem. BAMBY stands for:

Bran
And
Multiple vitamins and minerals
B Complex vitamins
Yogurt

While coarse bran, which is more effective than the finely ground, is easily available and inexpensive, it is for many people an inconvenient form of the fiber. I find people happier with the use of bran tablets. These are more expensive but not overly so, coming in 500-milligram tablets, two of which would roughly be equivalent to a teaspoonful of bran. A teaspoonful is the starting (test) amount, to establish tolerance. If intolerant of the fiber, or if you prove allergic to wheat bran, the trial stops at that point. If all is well, the dose is raised from two tablets to three daily, then to four, and perhaps even more. You know that you've reached the right amount when bowel movement is easy and effortless and, not incidentally, free of odor. The freedom from typical stool odor is a sign that stool transit time has been shortened to deprive the bowel bacteria of the opportunity to modify the chemicals in the food residues.

The multiple vitamins and minerals, and the separate B Complex supplement, provide factors which help digestion and utilization of food, and one which aids in stimulating peristalsis, the muscular movements which propel food residues through the gut. The yogurt helps by substituting friendly bacteria for undesirable types. Yogurt—which should be plain, not flavored or filled with sugar-saturated fruit—can be substituted for the skim milk permitted in the preceding menus. You can make yogurt inexpensively at home, and you will find yogurt makers—really, low-temperature hot plates—at the health food store and other stores. The quantity of yogurt needed significantly to alter the bacterial flora in some people may be too large, in terms of the amount of natural milk sugar yielded, considering the restrictions on sugar in the hypoglycemia diet. Yogurt may contain seven or eight grams of sugar per container, which, of course, has to be counted as part of the total carbohydrate content of the diet. You can overcome this problem by obtaining the bacteria from lactobacillus acidophilus tablets, available at the health food store.

Two warnings: in the first three weeks of high-fiber diet, flatulence often develops. It may appear again if you find it necessary to increase the dose of bran. *Don't* retain the gas, for the pressure on the gut is considerable, and may lead to diverticulosis. Treat the urge to vent gas as you would an urge for a bowel movement, and retire to the bathroom. Another problem is the penalty if you decide to stop the use of bran abruptly, in which case you may develop the grandfather of all cases of temporary constipation. Taper off, if you must—unless you've run into an allergy demanding quicker abstention. And mentioning allergy, reminds me to remind you that you must be sure that you're not allergic to any innovations in your menus or supplements.

Earlier, I referred to the diets—plural—for hypoglycemia. You can now understand why. There are those who will thrive on high protein, others who will do better on less. There will be those who will profit by restricting carbohydrate to sixty grams daily. Some will require less; some may need more, or may do better on a high carbohydrate intake, which for them may be fine—provided that the carbohydrates do not include sugar and aren't overprocessed. Experience for more than four decades tells me that the majority will do well on high protein and restricted carbohydrate, minus sugar. Some of these may require digestive aids—hydrochloric acid, for instance, the need for which *must* be established by your physician. Adverse effects may result from supplements of hydrochloric acid added to normal production. Pancreatic enzymes, bromelin—which comes from pineapple—and papain, from papaya, are examples of other enzyme digestive aids which are particularly helpful as the age of the user and his protein intake increase. Other variations on the diet are obvious: the use of bran and the BAMBY plan by those who need these adjuncts; and the use of vegetable oil to aid reducing, for those whose weight is complicating recovery from hypoglycemia, arthritis, or both.

I have a warning on my mind, as I close this section of the Appendix. Earlier, I named malnourishment as one of the potent causes of hypoglycemia. That malnourishment, nine times out of ten, involves eating Danish pastry rather than eggs for breakfast, luncheons of sandwiches with the bread outweighing the meat between the slices, skimpy dinners, and a plenitude of desserts, sweets, and bakery goods. All this spells a diet too low in protein and too high in carbohydrates. I think of this when I read books urging upon the arthritic and the hypoglycemic low protein diets, high in carbohydrate. It is a recommendation which repeats the pattern of eating that caused the troubles in the first place; the only change is in the substitution of whole grains for the processed starches and sugars. That, though, is small comfort to a body which has been deprived of protein. You might remember, as you read eulogies of low protein diets, what the word means. Protein means "of first importance."

THE CONSTRUCTIVE REDUCTION DIET

What if you have no allergies, hypoglycemia, or intolerance to nightshades, but you do have a bicycle tire (truck tire, zeppelin) at the midriff, and your doctor says arthritics profit by reducing?

In the diets for hypoglycemia, I included instructions for

converting the low carbohydrate into a reducing diet by the addition of vegetable oil. There are those who need a low-carbohydrate diet to lose weight because they have a metabolic quirk: when they eat starches and sugars, they turn them into fat with great efficiency, and they retain salt. When you reduce, you burn fat into water and a gas; if you retain salt, you retain the water and wind up not losing weight. There are millions of people, however, who don't need a low-carbohydrate diet to lose weight. All they require is a balanced diet which restricts calories. I call mine "The Constructive Reduction Diet" because it spurs you into burning fat, but doesn't do what fasting and severe diets do: make you burn tissues.

The supplements listed with this diet aren't optional. You must protect yourself against the reduction in vitamin-mineral intake when you cut your calories in half. And if you have problem areas where fat blithely clings to you, even though the scale says the lumps and bumps should be disappearing, there are supplements which sometimes will tend to distribute the fat deposits toward the normal. Read on; you are about to encounter menus which can be followed even when you're eating away from home, leaving you no excuse for failure.

In this diet, every effort has been made to keep vitamin-mineral intake as high as possible, protein intake more than adequate, with enough fat and carbohydrate to achieve a ratio which will not invite fatigue from ketosis.

Nonetheless, any diet below 2,400 calories risks vitamin-mineral deficiencies, no matter how careful the food selection, for this is a hazard inherent in reducing the gross intake of food, and the hazard increases as the calorie intake decreases. It is recommended that this diet, therefore, be supplemented with multiple vitamins and minerals, as a safeguard. You can do more than this, if you'd like to explore what supplements can do in helping you to distribute your weight loss more equitably, so that your problem areas may respond, and your face not sink in, leaving you looking cadaverous. To try to accomplish all this, add to your supplements lecithin, Vitamin B Complex (high in choline and inositol); and Vitamin E, in the form of mixed tocopherols. (And don't write to me to tell me I'm quoting Mary Ann Crenshaw, for it's the other way around: years ago, I performed controlled research in redistribution of body fat toward the normal, both by diet and by use of supplements. What you have just read, then, isn't theory: it derived from practical application, and it works beautifully in about one quarter of those who try it.)

By the code system employed, and the lists of foods, the need for set menus is eliminated and there is no need for counting calories. Thousands of overweight persons have followed this diet safely, without weakness, deficiency, or hunger.

Breakfast

1 serving of fruit
1 egg or egg substitute
½ slice (thin) whole wheat toast with ½ level teaspoonful butter.
1 glass of skim milk
1 cup of coffee or tea (optional)
    (no sugar; no cream or milk)

Lunch

1 helping of lean meat, fish, fowl, or meat substitute
1 vegetable from vegetable list A
1 salad (from salad list)
1 serving of fruit or dessert
1 glass of skim milk or buttermilk
1 cup of coffee or tea (optional)
    (no sugar, no cream or milk)

2

2

Dinner

1 cup of soup (optional)
1 helping of lean meat, fish, fowl, or meat substitute
2 vegetables from list A *plus* 1 from vegetable list B
or
1 vegetable from vegetable list A *plus* 1 from vegetable list
   B *plus* 1 helping of salad (from salad list)
1 portion of fruit or dessert
Coffee or tea (no sugar, no cream or milk)

Choose foods from the following lists:

Soup list

Consomme
Clear vegetable soup
Beef broth
Mutton broth
Chicken broth
Other clear soups
(No creamed soups, none with milk or content of vegeta-
   bles, meat, or cereals)

Fruit list

Orange (small)
Grapefruit (half, medium size)
Apple, (1, small)
Pineapple (2 average slices)
Peach (1)
Cantaloupe (1 half, medium size)
Melon (2-inch section of average-size melon)
Tangerine (1, large)
Berries (½ cup)
Apricots (2, medium size)

Grapes (12)
Cherries (10)
Pear (1, medium size)
Plums (2)
Nectarines (3)
Persimmon (½, small)
Fruit juices: grapefruit, orange (unsweetened) 6 ounces
(¾ water glass)

Meat list

Lean beefsteak (¼ pound, about 1 inch thick, 2½ inches
square)
Roast beef (2 slices, about 3 inches square, ¼ inch thick)
Beef liver (1 slice, 3 inches square, ½ inch thick)
Beef tongue (2 average slices)
Beef kidney (¼ pound)
Hamburger (¼ pound)
Calf's liver (¼ pound)
Lamb kidney (2, average size)
Lamb chop (1, about 2 inches square, ½ inch thick)
Roast lamb (1 slice, 3½ inches square, ¼ inch thick)
Mutton chop (2, medium size)
Boiled mutton (1 slice, 4 inches square, ½ inch thick)
Roast veal (1 slice, 3x2 inches, ¼ inch thick)
Veal cutlet (1, average size)
Veal kidney (2, average size)
Chicken, white meat (2 slices, 4 inches square, cut very
thin)
Chicken, broiler (½ medium size)
Chicken, gizzards (2, average size)
Chicken, livers (2 whole, medium size)

Fish list

Sea bass (¼ pound)

Bluefish (¼ pound)
Cod, fresh (¼ pound to ½ pound)
Cod, salt (¼ pound to ½ pound)
Flounder (¼ pound to ½ pound)
Haddock (¼ pound to ½ pound)
Halibut (¼ pound)
Kingfish (¼ pound)
Pike (¼ pound)
Porgy (¼ pound)
Red snapper (¼ pound)
Scallops (2/3 cup, raw measurement)
Shrimp (2/3 cup)
Smelt (¼ pound)
Weakfish (¼ pound)
Clams, round (10 to 12)
Crab meat (1 crab or ¾ cup flakes)
Lobster (½ small lobster or 1 cup flakes)
Mussels (4 large or 8 small)
Oysters (12 large)

Meat substitutes

Cottage cheese (2/3 cup)
Eggs (2)
Buttermilk (2 cups)
Whole milk (1 cup)
Skim milk (2 cups)

Eggs and egg substitutes

Prepare your egg in one of the following ways:
Plain omelet
Poached
Soft boiled
Hard boiled
Raw

Appendix

Substitutes for 1 egg

Cottage cheese (4 tablespoons)
Lamb chop (1 small, lean)
Lamb kidney (1)
Calf's liver (2 ounces)
Mutton chop (1 small, lean)
Buttermilk (1 glass)
Skim milk (1 glass)

Vegetable list A

Asparagus (fresh or canned: 8)
String beans (½ cup)
Wax beans (½ cup)
Beet greens (2 heaping tablespoons)
Broccoli (1 5-inch stalk)
Brussels sprouts (½ cup)
Cabbage, cooked (½ cup)
Cabbage, raw (¾ cup, shredded)
Cauliflower (½ cup)
Celery (5 stalks)
Chard (½ cup)
Chicory (½ cup)
Eggplant (½ cup)
Endive (10 medium stalks)
Green pepper (1, medium size)
Kohlrabi (2 heaping tablespoons)
Leek, chopped (1/3 cup)
Lettuce (10 leaves)
Radishes (5, medium size)
Sauerkraut (½ cup)
Spinach (½ cup)
Tomatoes, fresh (1)
Tomatoes, canned (½ cup)
Tomato juice: 4 ounces (½ cup)
Watercress (10 pieces)

Vegetable list B

Beets (2 heaping tablespoons)
Carrots (2 heaping tablespoons)
Chives (6)
Dandelion greens (3 heaping tablespoons)
Kale (2 heaping tablespoons)
Onion (1, small)
Parsnips (2 heaping tablespoons)
Peas (2 heaping tablespoons)
Pumpkin (3 heaping tablespoons)
Rutabaga (3 heaping tablespoons)
Squash (2 heaping tablespoons)
Turnips (2 heaping tablespoons)

Salads

Tossed greens
Watercress and lettuce
Radish and watercress
Celery and cabbage
Pimiento and greens
Stuffed tomato (cottage cheese, chopped celery)

(If butter is omitted from vegetables at lunch, 1 teaspoon of salad dressing may be used. Divide between lunch and dinner, if salads are eaten twice daily; use vinegar or lemon juice to augment.)

FOOD FAMILIES

Allergic individuals will find the following listings of food families* useful for two opposed purposes:

1. Allergy to one member of a food family indicates the strong possibility of allergy to other members. The listing is helpful, therefore, in avoiding unnecessary exposure to foods you are likely to find troublemakers. Remember though: "likely" doesn't mean *surely*. It simply raises a red flag, reading *caution*. Common sense tells you that a person strongly allergic to milk should be cautious with cheese and ice cream.
2. Conversely, the lists indicate safer areas. If you have absolutely no allergic reaction to one member of a food family, your chances of tolerating other foods in that group are obviously better.

In the first—alphabetical—list of foods you will find a number in front of each food. The second—numerical—list lets you track down that number, so that you can more easily identify other members of the family to which it belongs. If I may read your mind: yes, it's worth the trouble. Many failures in treatment of allergic individuals—arthritic or not—derive from their continuing to consume foods which are in the family of one to which they *know* they're allergic.

*Lists reproduced from *Coping with Your Allergies* by Natalie Golos and Frances Golos Golbitz with Frances Spatz Leighton. Copyright © 1979 by Frances Golos Golbitz. Reprinted by permission of Simon & Schuster, a Division of Gulf & Western Corporation.

List 1: Food Families (Alphabetical)

A

81	abalone
80	absinthe
41	acacia (gum)
46	acerola
79	acorn squash
1	agar-agar
12	agave
98	albacore
41	alfalfa
1	Algae
63	allspice
40b	almond
11	*Aloe vera*
54	althea root
12	Amaryllis Family
94	amberjack
86	American eel
117	amphibians
5	anchovy
63	angelica
65	anise
38	annatto
136	antelope
40a	apple
73	apple mint
40b	apricot
47	arrowroot, Brazilian (tapioca)
9	arrowroot (*Colocasia*)
17	arrowroot, East Indian (*Curcuma*)
19	Arrowroot Family
13	arrowroot (Figi)
4	arrowroot, Florida (*Zamia*)
19	arrowroot (*Maranta* starch)
16	arrowroot (*Musa*)
18	arrowroot, Queensland
80	artichoke flour
9	Arum Family
11	asparagus
2	*Aspergillus*
34	avocado

B

2	baker's yeast
6	bamboo shoots
16	banana
16	Banana Family
46	Barbados cherry
6	barley
73	basil
114	bass (black)
113	bass (yellow)
53	basswood
34	bay leaf
41	bean
132	bear
66	bearberry
24	Beech Family
137	beef
28	beet
7	bell pepper
73	bergamot

191

Appendix

80 celtuce	55 cocoa butter
9 ceriman	8 coconut
80 chamomile	79 cocozelle
52 champagne	87 cod (scrod)
28 chard	76 coffee
79 chayote	55 cola nut
40b cherry	36 collards
65 chervil	80 coltsfoot
24 chestnut	36 colza shoots
73 chia seed	71 comfrey
124 chicken	80 Composite Family
41 chickpea	5 Conifer Family
67 chicle	65 coriander
80 chicory	6 corn
71 chili pepper	78 corn-salad
36 Chinese cabbage	80 costmary
56 Chinese gooseberry	54 cottonseed
14 Chinese potato	41 coumarin
79 Chinese preserving melon	36 couve tronchuda
7 Chinese water chestnut	41 cowpea
24 chinquapin	82 crab
11 chives	40a crabapple
55 chocolate	66 cranberry
111 chub	114 crappie
7 chufa	82 crayfish
40a cider	52 cream of tartar
34 cinnamon	79 crenshaw melon
1 citric acid	96 croaker
45 citron	79 crookneck squash
6 citronella	79 cucumber
45 Citrus Family	65 cumin
81 clam	36 curly cress
73 clary	39 currant
63 clove	79 cushaw squash
41 clover	81 cusk
55 cocoa	32 custard-apple

193

Appendix

121	goose
39	gooseberry
28	Goosefoot Family
65	gotu kola
79	Gourd Family
6	graham flour
58	granadilla
52	grape
52	Grape Family
45	grapefruit
6	Grass Family
61	grenadine
6	grits
74	ground cherry
7	groundnut
91	grouper
123	grouse (ruffed)
63	guava
125	guinea fowl
41	gum acacia
41	gum tragacanth

H

87	haddock
87	hake
103	halibut
101	harvest fish
23	hazelnut
22	heartnut
66	Heath Family
54	hibiscus
22	hickory nut
134	hog
49	Holly Family
6	hominy
79	honeydew

77	Honeysuckle Family
25	hop
73	horehound
133	horse
36	horseradish
3	horsetail
3	Horsetail Family
79	Hubbard squash
6	huckleberry
73	hyssop

I

15	Iris Family
1	Irish moss

J

68	Japanese persimmon
80	Jerusalem artichoke
41	jicama
5	juniper

K

68	kaki
36	kale
1	kelp
41	kidney bean
56	kiwi berry
36	kohlrabi
45	kumquat

L

137	lamb
28	lamb's-quarters
34	Laurel Family
73	lavender

43 nasturtium
43 Nasturtium Family
41 navy bean
40 nectarine
29 New Zealand spinach
97 northern scup
33 nutmeg
33 Nutmeg Family
2 nutritional yeast

O

6 oat
6 outmeal
88 ocean catfish
102 ocean perch
23 oil of birch
54 okra
69 olive
69 Olive Family
11 onion
128 opossum
45 orange
20 Orchid Family
73 oregano
15 orris root
42 oxalis
42 Oxalis Family
81 oyster
80 oyster plant

P

8 palm cabbage
8 Palm Family
59 papaya

59 Papaya Family
74 paprika
62 paradise nut
65 parsley
65 parsnip
123 partridge
58 Passion Flower Family
58 passion fruit
6 patent flour
79 pattypan squash
32 pawpaw
41 pea
40 peach
124 peafowl
41 peanut
40 pear
22 pecan
40 pectin
75 Pedalium Family
73 pennyroyal
74 pepino
74 pepper
21 peppercorn
21 Pepper Family
73 peppermint
102 perch (ocean)
113 perch (white)
115 perch (yellow)
79 Persian melon
68 persimmon
124 pheasant
109 pickerel
122 pigeon (squab)
30 pigweed
109 pike

Appendix

8	sago starch
99	sailfish
106	salmon species
80	salsify
80	santolina
67	Sapodilla Family
62	Sapucaya Family
62	sapucaya nut
11	sarsaparilla
34	sassafras
115	sauger (perch)
73	savory
39	Saxifrage Family
81	scallop
80	scolymus
80	scorzonera
91	Sea Bass Family
27	sea grape
84	sea herring
96	sea trout
1	seaweed
7	Sedge Family
41	senna
75	sesame
105	shad (roe)
11	shallot
3	shavegrass
137	sheep
82	shrimp
90	silver perch
90	silverside
98	skipjack
40	sloe
108	smelt
81	snail
51	Soapberry Family

11	soap plant
103	sole
6	sorghum
27	sorrel
80	southernwood
41	soybean
41	soy products
73	spearmint
28	spinach
96	spot
96	spotted sea trout
47	Spurge Family
79	squash
81	squid
130	squirrel
55	Sterculia Family
40	strawberry
41	string bean
110	sucker
28	sugar beet
6	sugar cane
73	summer savory
114	sunfish
80	sunflower seed products
36	swede
65	sweet cicely
6	sweet corn
74	sweet pepper
70	sweet potato
100	swordfish

T

13	Tacca Family
75	tahini
41	tamarind
28	tampala

Appendix

45	tangelo
45	tangerine
80	tansy
47	tapioca
9	taro
80	tarragon
57	tea
57	Tea Family
12	tequila
120	terrapin
73	thyme
92	tilefish
74	tobacco
74	tomatillo
74	tomato
41	tonka bean
74	tree tomato
6	triticale
106	trout species
2	truffle
98	tuna
79	turban squash
103	turbot
126	turkey
17	turmeric
36	turnip
120	turtle species

U

36	upland cress

V

78	Valerian Family
20	vanilla
80	vegetable spaghetti

135	venison
71	Verbena Family
40	vinegar

W

115	walleye
22	Walnut Family
36	watercress
79	watermelon
96	weakfish
19	West Indian arrowfoot
131	whale
9	wheat
9	wheat germ
90	whitebait
107	whitefish
21	white pepper
113	white perch
6	wild rice
40	wineberry
52	wine vinegar
23	wintergreen
73	winter savory
80	witloof
76	woodruff
80	wormwood

Y

14	yam
14	Yam Family
14	yampi
80	yarrow
9	yautia
113	yellow bass

Appendix

List 2: Food Families (Numerical)

Plant

1 Algae
   agar-agar
   carrageen (Irish moss)
   *dulse
   kelp (seaweed)
2 Fungi
   baker's yeast ("Red Star")
   brewer's or nutritional
      yeast
   mold (in certain cheeses)
   citric acid (*Aspergillus*)
   morel
   mushroom
   puffball
   truffle
3 Horsetail Family,
   Equisetaceae
   *shavegrass (horsetail)
4 Cycad Family, *Cycadaceae*
   Florida arrowroot (*Zamia*)
5 Conifer Family, *Coniferae*
   *juniper (gin)
   pine nut (pinon, pinyon)
6 Grass Family, *Gramineae*
   barley
      malt
      maltose
   bamboo shoots
   corn (mature)
      corn meal

corn oil
cornstarch
corn sugar
corn syrup
hominy grits
lemon grass
millet
oat
   oatmeal
popcorn
rice
   rice flour
rye
sorghum grain
   syrup
sugar cane
   cane sugar
   molasses
   raw sugar
sweet corn
triticale
wheat
   bran (semolina)
   bulgur
   flour
      gluten
      graham
      patent
      whole wheat
   wheat germ

*One or more plant parts (leaf, root, seed, etc.) used as a beverage.

wild rice
7 Sedge Family, *Cyperaceae*
Chinese water chestnut
chufa (groundnut)
8 Palm Family, *Palmaceae*
coconut
coconut meal
coconut oil
date
date sugar
palm cabbage
sago starch (*Metroxylon*)
9 Arum Family, *Araceae*
ceriman (*Monstera*)
dasheen (*Colocasia*)
arrowroot
taro (*Colocasia*) arrowroot
poi
malanga (*Xanthosoma*)
yautia (*Xanthosoma*)
10 Pineapple Family,
Bromeliaceae
pineapple
11 Lily Family, *Liliaceae*
Aloe vera
asparagus
chives
garlic
leek
onion
ramp
*sarsaparilla
shallot
yucca (soap plant)
12 Amaryllis Family,
Amaryllidaceae
agave
mescal, pulque, and
tequila
13 Tacca Family, *Taccaceae*
Fiji arrowroot (*Tacca*)
14 Yam Family, *Dioscoreaceae*
Chinese potato (yam)
ñame (yampi)

15 Iris Family, *Iridaceae*
orris root (scent)
saffron (*Crocus*)
16 Banana Family, *Musaceae*
arrowroot (Musa)
banana
plantain
17 Ginger Family,
Zingiberaceae
cardamom
East Indian arrowroot
(*Curcuma*)
ginger
turmeric
18 Canna Family, *Cannaceae*
Queensland arrowroot
19 Arrowroot Family,
Marantaceae
arrowroot (*Maranta*
starch)
20 Orchid Family, *Orchidaceae*
vanilla
21 Pepper Family, *Piperaceae*
peppercorn (*Piper*)
22 Walnut Family,
Juglandaceae
black walnut
butternut
English walnut
heartnut
hickory nut
pecan
23 Birch Family, *Betulaceae*
filbert (hazelnut)
oil of birch (wintergreen)
(some wintergreen
flavor is
methyl salicylate)
24 Beech Family, *Fagaceae*
chestnut
chinquapin
25 Mulberry Family, *Moraceae*
breadfruit
fig

*One or more plant parts (leaf, root, seed, etc.) used as a beverage.

Appendix

*hop
mulberry
26 Protea Family, *Proteaceae*
    macadamia (Queensland
    nut)
27 Buckwheat Family,
    Polygonaceae
    buckwheat
    garden sorrel
    rhubarb
    sea grape
28 Goosefoot Family,
    Chenopodiaceae
    beet
    chard
    lamb's-quarters
    spinach
    sugar beet
    tampala
29 Carpetweed Family,
    Aizoaceae
    New Zealand spinach
30 Purslane Family,
    Portulacaceae
    pigweed (purslane)
31 Buttercup Family,
    Ranunculaceae
    *golden seal
32 Custard-Apple Family
    Annona species
    custard-apple
    papaw (pawpaw)
33 Nutmeg Family,
    Myristicaceae
    nutmeg
    mace
34 Laurel Family, *Lauraceae*
    avocado
    bay leaf
    cassia bark
    cinnamon
    *sassafras
      filé (powdered leaves)
35 Poppy Family, *Papaveraceae*
    poppyseed

36 Mustard Family, *Cruciferae*
    broccoli
    Brussels sprouts
    cabbage
    cauliflower
    Chinese cabbage
    collards
    colza shoot
    couve tronchuda
    curly cress
    horseradish
    kale
    kohlrabi
    mustard greens
    mustard seed
    radish
    rape
    rutabaga (swede)
    turnip
    upland cress
    watercress
37 Caper Family, *Capparidaceae*
    caper
38 Bixa Family, *Bixaceae*
    annatto (natural yellow
    dye)
39 Saxifrage Family,
    Saxifragaceae
    currant
    gooseberry
40 Rose Family, *Rosaceae*
a. pomes
    apple
      cider, vinegar
      pectin
    crabapple
    loquat
    pear
    quince
    *rosehips
b. stone fruits
    almond
    apricot
    cherry
    peach (nectarine)

*One or more plant parts (leaf, root, seed, etc.) used as a beverage.

plum (prune)
sloe
c. berries
blackberry
boysenberry
dewberry
loganberry
longberry
youngberry
*raspberry (leaf)
black raspberry
red raspberry
purple raspberry
*strawberry (leaf)
wineberry
d. herb
burnet (cucumber flavor)
41 Legume Family,
Leguminosae
*alfalfa (sprouts)
beans
fava
lima
mung (sprouts)
navy
string (kidney)
black-eyed pea (cowpea)
*carob
carob syrup
chickpea (garbanzo)
*fenugreek
gum acaia
gum tragacanth
jicama
kudzu
lentil
*licorice
pea
peanut
peanut oil
*red clover
*senna
soybean
lecithin
soy flour

soy grits
soy milk
soy oil
tamarind
tonka bean
coumarin
42 Oxalis Family, Oxalidaceae
carambola
oxalis
43 Nasturtium Family,
Tropaeolaceae
nasturtium
44 Flax Family, Linaceae
*flaxseed
45 Rue (Citrus) Family,
Rutaceae
citron
grapefruit
kumquat
lemon
lime
murcot
orange
pummelo
tangelo
tangerine
46 Malpighia Family,
Malpighiacea
acerola (Barbados cherry)
47 Spurge Family,
Euphorbiaceae
cassava or yuca (Manihot)
cassava meal
tapioca (Brazilian
arrowroot)
castor bean
castor oil
48 Cashew Family,
Anacardiaceae
cashew
mango
pistachio
poison ivy
poison oak
poison sumac

*One or more plant parts (leaf, root, seed, etc.) used as a beverage.

Appendix

49 Holly Family, *Aquifoliaceae*
    maté (yerba maté)
50 Maple Family
    maple sugar
    maple syrup
51 Soapberry Family,
    Sapindaceae
    litchi (lychee)
52 Grape Family, *Vitaceae*
    grape
      brandy
      champagne
      cream of tartar
      dried "currant"
      raisin
      wine
      wine vinegar
    muscadine
53 Linden Family, *Tiliaceae*
    *basswood (linden)
54 Mallow Family, *Malvaceae*
    *althea root
    cottonseed oil
    *hibiscus (roselle)
    okra
55 Sterculia Family,
    Sterculiaceae
    *chocolate (cacao)
    *cocoa
    cola nut
56 Dillenia Family, *Dilleniaceae*
    Chinese gooseberry (kiwi
    berry)
57 Tea Family, *Theaceae*
    *tea
58 Passion Flower Family,
    Passifloraceae
    granadilla (passion fruit)
59 Papaya Family, *Caricaeae*
    papaya
60 Cactus Family, *Cactaceae*
    prickly pear
61 Pomegranate Family,
    Puniceae
    pomegranate

    grenadine
62 Sapucaya Family,
    Lecythidaceae
    Brazil nut
    sapucaya nut (paradise
    nut)
63 Myrtle Family, *Myrtaceae*
    allspice (Pimenta)
    clove
    *eucalyptus
    guava
64 Ginseng Family, *Sraliaceae*
    *American ginseng
    *Chinese ginseng
65 Carrot Family, *Umbelliferae*
    angelica
    anise
    caraway
    carrot
      carrot syrup
    celeriac (celery root)
    celery
      *seed and leaf
    chervil
    coriander
    cumin
    dill
      dill seed
    *fennel
      finocchio or Florence
      fennel
    *gotu kola
    *lovage
    *parsley
    parsnip
    sweet cicely
66 Heath Family, *Ericaceae*
    *bearberry
    *blueberry
    cranberry
    *huckleberry
67 Sapodilla Family, *Sapotaceae*
    chicle (chewing gum)
68 Ebony Family, *Ebonaceae*
    American persimmon

*One or more plant parts (leaf, root, seed, etc.) used as a beverage.

206

Food Families

kaki (Japanese
persimmon)
69 Olive Family, *Oleaceae*
olive (green or ripe)
olive oil
70 Morning Glory Family,
Convolvulaceae
sweet potato
71 Borage Family, *Boraginaceae*
(Herbs)
borage
*comfrey (leaf and root)
72 Verbena Family,
Verbenaceae
*lemon verbena
73 Mint Family, *Labiatae*
(Herbs)
apple mint
basil
bergamot
*catnip
*chia seed
clary
*dittany
*horehound
*hyssop
lavender
*lemon balm
marjoram
oregano
*pennyroyal
*peppermint
rosemary
sage
*spearmint
summer savory
thyme
winter savory
74 Potato Family, *Solanaceae*
eggplant
ground cherry
pepino
(melon pear)
pepper (Capsicum)
bell, sweet

cayenne
chili
paprika
pimiento
potato
tobacco
tomatillo
tomato
tree tomato
75 Pedalium Family, *Pedaliaceae*
sesame seed
sesame oil
76 Madder Family, *Rubieceae*
*coffee
woodruff
77 Honeysuckle Family,
Caprifoliaceae
elderberry
elderberry flowers
78 Valerian Family,
Valerianaceae
corn salad (fetticus)
79 Gourd Family,
Cucurbitaceae
chayote
Chinese preserving melon
cucumber
gherkin
loofah (*Luffa*) (vegetable
sponge)
muskmelons
cantaloupe
casaba
crenshaw
honeydew
Persian melon
pumpkin
pumpkin seed and meal
squashes
acorn
buttercup
butternut
Boston marrow
caserta
cocozelle

*One or more plant parts (leaf, root, seed, etc.) used as a beverage.

Appendix

crookneck and
  straightneck
cushaw
golden nugget
Hubbard varieties
pattypan
turban
vegetable spaghetti
zucchini
watermelon
80 Composite Family,
  Compositae
  *boneset
  *burdock root
  cardoon
  chamomile
  *chicory
  coltsfoot
  costmary
  dandelion
  endive
  escarole
  globe artichoke

*goldenrod
Jerusalem artichoke
  artichoke flour
lettuce
  celtuce
pyrethrum
romaine
safflower oil
salsify (oyster plant)
santolina (herb)
scolymus (Spanish oyster
  plant)
scorzonera (black salsify)
southernwood
sunflower
  sunflower seed, meal
  and oil
tansy (herb)
tarragon (herb)
witloof chicory (French
  endive)
wormwood (absinthe)
*yarrow

Animal

81 Mollusks
  Gastropods
    abalone
    snail
  Cephalopod
    squid
  Pelecypods
    clam
    cockles
    mussel
    oyster
    scallop
82 Crustaceans
  crab
  crayfish
  lobster
  prawn
  shrimp
83 Fishes (saltwater)

84 Herring Family
  menhaden
  pilchard (sardine)
  sea herring
85 Anchovy Family
  anchovy
86 Eel Family
  American eel
87 Codfish Family
  cod (scrod)
  cusk
  haddock
  hake
  pollack
88 Sea Catfish Family
  ocean catfish
89 Mullet Family
  mullet
90 Silverside Family

*One or more plant parts (leaf, root, seed, etc.) used as a beverage.

silverside (whitebait)
91 Sea Bass Family
grouper
sea bass
92 Tilefish Family
tilefish
93 Bluefish Family
bluefish
94 Jack Family
amberjack
pompano
yellow jack
95 Dolphin Family
dolphin
96 Croaker Family
croaker
drum
sea trout
silver perch
spot
weakfish (spotted sea
trout)
97 Porgy Family
northern scup (porgy)
98 Mackerel Family
albacore
bonito
mackerel
skipjack
tuna
99 Marlin Family
marlin
sailfish
100 Swordfish Family
swordfish
101 Harvestfish Family
butterfish
harvestfish
102 Scorpionfish Family
rosefish (ocean perch)
103 Flounder Family
dab
flounder
halibut
plaice
sole

turbot
104 Fishes (freshwater)
Sturgeon Family
sturgeon (caviar)
105 Herring Family
shad (roe)
106 Salmon Family
salmon species
trout species
107 Whitefish Family
whitefish
108 Smelt Family
smelt
109 Pike Family
muskellunge
pickerel
pike
110 Sucker Family
buffalofish
sucker
111 Minnow Family
carp
chub
112 Catfish Family
catfish species
113 Bass Family
white perch
yellow bass
114 Sunfish Family
black bass species
sunfish species
pumpkinseed
crappie
115 Perch Family
sauger
walleye
yellow perch
116 Croaker Family
freshwater drum
117 Amphibians
Frog Family
frog (frogs' legs)
118 Reptiles
119 Snake Family
rattlesnake
120 Turtle Family

Appendix

SOURCES OF PROFESSIONAL HELP

On every medical diploma, the medical man is described as "physician and surgeon." Yet every layman knows that only specially trained and qualified physicians are described as surgeons, and permitted to perform operations. By the same token, the ethical physician will disqualify himself if you ask him for services beyond the range of his training and competence. The internist will send you to a specialist for X-raying and interpretation of the results. For complicated gynecological problems, he will refer you to a gynecologist; for psychiatric problems, to a psychiatrist; for a broken bone, to an orthopedist; and for periodontal disease, to a dentist qualified in that type of treatment. But when you ask a physician for reference to a medical nutritionist, too often he reacts as though you were challenging his prerogatives and competence in the entire field of medicine. The fact is, though, that a majority of medical schools teach no nutrition. Some make it an optional course—which students interpret as meaning it isn't important. And in the list of continuing medical education courses, in the 1980 schedule of the American Medical Association, among hundreds of subjects, nutrition isn't even mentioned. All this adds up to a simple statement: you are entitled to a consultation with a specialist. This doesn't mean that you must part company with your present physician, and it certainly doesn't mean that he, in turn, should be outraged and, as has sometimes happened, refuse to continue as your personal doctor.

I have just given you my reasons for supplying you with lists of medical societies devoted to holistic medicine, preventive medicine, and nutrition. In querying these organizations for referral to a medical nutritionist to treat your arthritis, you must remember that within such societies, there are represented many different types of specialties in medicine. There are pediatricians who practice nutrition, and psychiatrists who use it instead of couch, conversation, and calmative drugs. There are proctologists who employ nutrition as part of their systems of treatment, and gynecologists who do, too. You must therefore specify very clearly what type of medical service you wish. If you ask to be referred to rheumatologists (arthritis specialists) who treat such disorders nutritionally, you may find that a few are so listed with the particular society. You are more likely to be referred, however, to a medical nutritionist who is actually a general practitioner, but who does treat rheumatic and arthritic disorders with nutrition.

Another admonition: don't expect to be referred to a practitioner on your street or, for that matter, in your city. Every day, more and more physicians move into holistic medicine and nutrition, but ours is a large country, and a few thousand physicians, gratifying as the numbers are, are spread thin. If you are determined to find genuine help in nutrition, rather than palliative drug therapy, stick to your guns.

Practitioners who treat hypoglycemia, who are aware of the role of the total environment in allergies, and who are sensitive to the importance of nutrition as an aid in the treatment of arthritic diseases may be members of the following medical societies:

The International Academy of Preventive Medicine, 10409 Town and Country Way, Suite 200, Houston, TX 77024. Ask for their directory, and enclose fifteen cents in stamps, as a minimum, or enclose one dollar as the actual cost of their providing you with their directory, which lists hundreds of practitioners from coast to coast. Neither postage nor the one dollar contribution is mandatory.

International Academy of Metabology, care of Dr. Arthur L. Kaslow, 2235 Castillo Street, Suite B, Medical Foundation, Santa Barbara, CA 93105. Mostly California practitioners, but some in other areas.

International College of Applied Nutrition, Box 386, La Habra, CA 90631. Membership mostly in California, but some practitioners in other areas.

American Academy of Medical Preventics. 8383 Wilshire Boulevard, Beverly Hills, CA 90211. This group is devoted primarily to chelation, a method of treating cardiovascular diseases which substitutes in appropriate cases for bypass surgery. It is also used for impaired circulation in diabetes and arthritis. Nutrition is an important adjunct to this treatment, and most of the members are thereby practicing holistic medicine and nutrition, coupled with prevention.

Society for Clinical Ecology, care of Robert Collier, M.D., Secretary, 4045 Wadsworth Boulevard, Wheat Ridge, CO 80033. Diagnostic services and treatment for allergy in terms of the total internal and external environments. This differs thereby from conventional allergy practice, and may be much more suited to the needs of the allergic arthritic, since allergy in arthritis is an entity neglected both by conventional allergists and by rheumatologists.

The Huxley Institute, 1114 First Avenue, New York, NY 10021. Distributes information on both orthomolecular psychiatry and medicine. Maintains a referral list of physicians who practice in this field. You should make it clear, in your inquiry, that you are seeking nutritional help for arthritis.

Index

Index

Index

Index

Pellagra, 112
Penicillamine, 9, 32, 69
Penicillin, 100
Peppers, avoidance of, 18-46, 107
Pesticides, 62, 72
Pfeiffer, Dr. Carl C., 98, 139, 141
Phlebitis, 145
Physiotherapy, 17, 103
Pituitary gland, 96, 136, 143, 144, 164
Pizza, 22, 37
Placebo effect, 133, 141
POTABA, 164
Potassium, 13, 88, 149, 151, 154-55
Potato chips, 22, 45
Potato salad, 23, 28
Potatoes, white, avoidance of, 18-46, 107
PPET foods, avoidance of, 18-46
Price, Dr. Weston A., 74
Pritikin, Nathan, 74
Professional help, sources of, 211-213
Progesterone, 154
Prostate gland, 148
Protein, 100, 182
  predigested, 64
Pulse-rate method of diagnosing allergies, 49, 53-55, 56
Pulse Test, The (Coca), 54
Pyridoxin, 111, 151-54, 160, 165

Q

Questionnaire, no-nightshade diet, 26

R

Ragweed, 58
Raisins, 155
Randolph, Dr. Theron, 59, 60
RAST test, 52, 57
Reduction diet, constructive, 182-89
Rheumatic fever, 74, 91, 100, 102
Rheumatism, 152
Rheumatoid arthritis, 18, 47, 59, 66, 67, 69, 70, 73, 74, 79, 90-111, 126, 129, 139, 140, 159, 165
Rhubarb, 43
Riboflavin, 120
Ringsdorf, Dr. W. M., Jr., 139 fn.
Rinkel test, 52, 57
Rotation diet, 55-56, 61
Royal jelly, 97, 98
Rutabaga, 138
Rutin, 68, 160

S

Saccharin, 172
Salicylic acid, 100
Salt, 138, 154
Schizophrenia, 112, 113, 148
"Scratch" test, 50, 52
Scurvy, 98, 99
Selenium, 145, 155-56, 163
Shellfish, 142
Slow stool transit time, 179-80
Society for Clinical Ecology, 213
Solanine, 22, 44-45
Soy products, 58, 138
Spies, Dr. Tom, 12, 14, 112
Spinach, 43
Stefansson, Vilhjalmur, 167
Still's disease, 74
Stroud, Dr. Robert, 59
Stress, 18, 19, 79, 91, 97-99, 100, 101, 161
  heredity and, 169
Sublingual test, 52, 57
Sucrose, 171
Sugar, 73, 75, 76, 79, 80, 82, 89, 92, 171-73
Supernutrition, 167

T

Tea, 43, 172, 173
  herb, 30, 58, 173
Tendonitis, 18, 29, 30, 59
Therapeutic diagnosis, 56, 108
Thiamin, 105
Thiamine, 120, 121
Thrombophlebitis, 145
Thrombosis, 145
Thymus gland, 93, 95, 165
Thyroid gland, 136-39, 141, 146
Tobacco, 26, 40, 107
Tocopherols, 95, 103, 110, 145-46, 147, 160, 165, 184
Tomatoes, avoidance of, 18-46, 51, 107,
Tonsils, 92
Torula yeast, 163
Tuttle, Dr. Esther, 13, 97

U

Ulcers, 154
United Airlines, 75

V

Vegetarianism, 72, 104, 167